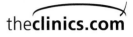

NURSING CLINICS OF NORTH AMERICA

Vulnerable Populations

GUEST EDITORS
Marcia Stanhope, RN, DSN, FAAN
Lisa M. Turner, MSN, APRN, BC
Peggy Riley, RN, MSN

CONSULTING EDITOR
Suzanne S. Prevost, PhD, RN

September 2008 • Volume 43 • Number 3

SAUNDERS

An Imprint of Elsevier, Inc.
PHILADELPHIA   LONDON   TORONTO   MONTREAL   SYDNEY   TOKYO

W.B. SAUNDERS COMPANY

A Division of Elsevier Inc.

1600 John F. Kennedy Blvd., Suite 1800, Philadelphia, PA 19103-2899

http://www.theclinics.com

NURSING CLINICS OF NORTH AMERICA
September 2008
Editor: Ali Gavenda

Volume 43, Number 3
ISSN 0029-6465
ISBN-13: 978-1-4160-6324-7
ISBN-10: 1-4160-6324-2

Nursing Clinics of North America (ISSN 0029-6465) is published quarterly by Elsevier Inc., 360 Park Avenue South, New York, NY 10010-1710. Months of issue are March, June, September, and December. Business and Editorial Offices: 1600 John F. Kennedy Blvd., Suite 1800, Philadelphia, PA 19103-2899. Customer Service Office: 6277 Sea Harbor Drive, Orlando, FL 32887-4800. Periodicals postage paid at New York, NY and additional mailing offices. Subscription price per year is, $123.00 (US individuals), $242.00 (US institutions), $198.00 (international individuals), $290.00 (international institutions), $170.00 (Canadian individuals), $290.00 (Canadian institutions), $65.00 (US students), and $100.00 (international students). To receive student/resident rate, orders must be accompanied by name of affiliated institution, date of term, and the signature of program/residency coordinator on institution letterhead. Orders will be billed at individual rate until proof of status is received. Foreign air speed delivery is included in all *Clinics* subscription prices. All prices are subject to change without notice. **POSTMASTER:** Send address changes to *Nursing Clinics*, Elsevier Periodicals Customer Service, 6277 Sea Harbor Drive, Orlando, FL 32887-4800. **Customer Service: 1-800-654-2452 (US). From outside the United States, call 1-407-563-6020. Fax: 1-407-363-9661. E-mail: JournalsCustomerService-usa@elsevier.com.**

Nursing Clinics of North America is covered in *EMBASE/Excerpta Medica, MEDLINE/PubMed (Index Medicus), Social Sciences Citation Index, Current Contents, ASCA, Cumulative Index to Nursing, RNdex Top 100,* and *Allied Health Literature and International Nursing Index (INI).*

Printed in the United States of America.

CONSULTING EDITOR

SUZANNE S. PREVOST, PhD, RN, Nursing Professor and National HealthCare Chair of Excellence, School of Nursing, Middle Tennessee State University, Murfreesboro, Tennessee

GUEST EDITORS

MARCIA STANHOPE, RN, DSN, FAAN, Professor and Good Samaritan Endowed Chair in Community Health Nursing, College of Nursing, University of Kentucky, Lexington, Kentucky

LISA M. TURNER, MSN, APRN, BC, Research Intern, Good Samaritan Nursing Center, College of Nursing, University of Kentucky, Lexington, Kentucky

PEGGY RILEY, RN, MSN, Extension Health Specialist for Nursing, Health Education through Extension Leadership Program, College of Agriculture and College of Nursing, University of Kentucky, Lexington, Kentucky

CONTRIBUTORS

SETH ALLCORN, PhD, Vice President for Business and Finance, The University of New England, Biddeford, Maine

DEBRA GAY ANDERSON, PhD, APRN, BC, Associate Professor, College of Nursing, University of Kentucky, Lexington, Kentucky

MELISSA D. AVERY, PhD, CNM, FACNM, Associate Professor and Chair, Child and Family Health Cooperative, University of Minnesota School of Nursing, Minneapolis, Minnesota

MARY BENBENEK, MS, RN, FNP, PNP, Clinical Assistant Professor, University of Minnesota School of Nursing, Minneapolis, Minnesota

LYNDA BILLINGS, MFA, Assistant Professor, School of Nursing, Texas Tech University–Health Sciences Center, Lubbock, Texas

MALLORY BOYLAN, PhD, Professor, Nutrition and Dietetics, College of Human Sciences, Texas Tech University, Lubbock, Texas

LINDA BULLOCK, PhD, RN, FAAN, Professor, Sinclair School of Nursing, University of Missouri–Columbia, Columbia, Missouri

CHIUNGHSIN CHANG, MS, Doctoral Student, Human Development and Family Studies, University of Missouri–Columbia, Columbia, Missouri

PAMELA D. CONNOR, PhD, Professor, Department of Preventive Medicine, College of Medicine, The University of Tennessee Health Science Center, Memphis, Tennessee

PATRICIA D. CUNNINGHAM, DNSc, APRN-PMH, FNP-BC, College of Nursing, The University of Tennessee Health Science Center, Memphis, Tennessee

DEBORAH D. DANNER, PhD, Sanders-Brown Center on Aging, Alzheimer's Disease Center; and Department of Preventive Medicine and Environmental Health, College of Public Health, University of Kentucky, Lexington, Kentucky

TONYA EDDY, MS(N), RN, Instructor of Clinical Nursing and Doctoral Student, Sinclair School of Nursing, University of Missouri–Columbia, Columbia, Missouri

M. CHRISTINA ESPERAT, PhD, RN, FAAN, Associate Dean for Research and Practice and CH Foundation Regents Professor in Rural Heath Disparities, School of Nursing, Texas Tech University–Health Sciences Center, Lubbock, Texas

DU FENG, PhD, Associate Professor, Human Development and Family Studies, College of Human Sciences, Texas Tech University, Lubbock, Texas

BELINDA FLEMING, PhD(c), MSN, FNP-BC, College of Nursing, The University of Tennessee Health Science Center, Memphis, Tennessee

VICTORIA FLORIANI, RN, CPNP, APRN-BC, Department of Family Health Care Nursing, University of California, San Francisco, California

MARGARET T. HARTIG, PhD, PFNP, FNP-BC, Professor and Chair, Primary Care and Public Health, College of Nursing, The University of Tennessee Health Science Center, Memphis, Tennessee

JOANNA HUDSON, RN, Sanders-Brown Center on Aging, Alzheimer's Disease Center, University of Kentucky, Lexington, Kentucky

PEACE JESSA, MD, Sanders-Brown Center on Aging, Alzheimer's Disease Center; Department of Preventive Medicine and Environmental Health, College of Public Health, University of Kentucky, Lexington, Kentucky

CHRISTINE KENNEDY, RN, CPNP, PhD, FAAN, Professor, Department of Family Health Care Nursing, University of California, San Francisco, California

ERIN KILBURN, MS(N), RN, Instructor of Clinical Nursing and Doctoral Student, Sinclair School of Nursing, University of Missouri–Columbia, Columbia, Missouri

MARY LASHLEY, PhD, RN, APRN, BC, Professor, Community Health Nursing, Towson University, Towson, Maryland

YONDELL MASTEN, RNC, PhD, WHNP, CNS, Professor and Associate Dean for Outcomes Management and Evaluation, School of Nursing, Texas Tech University–Health Sciences Center, Lubbock, Texas

CAROL O'BOYLE, PhD, RN, Associate Professor, University of Minnesota School of Nursing, Minneapolis, Minnesota

BARBARA PENCE, PhD, Associate Vice President for Research and Associate Dean for Graduate School of Biomedical Sciences, Texas Tech University–Health Sciences Center, Lubbock, Texas

JEANNE PFEIFFER, RN, MPH, CIC, Clinical Assistant Professor and MERET Grant Coordinator, University of Minnesota School of Nursing, Minneapolis, Minnesota

ROBBIE PREPAS, CNM, MN, JD, Adjunct Professor, UCLA-Harbor Medical Center Nurse Practitioner Program, Laguna Beach, California

PEGGY RILEY, RN, MSN, Extension Health Specialist for Nursing, Health Education through Extension Leadership Program, College of Agriculture and College of Nursing, University of Kentucky, Lexington, Kentucky

LOIS R. ROBLEY, PhD, RN, Professor of Ethics and Assistant Director, Siegel Institute for Leadership, Ethics, and Character, Kennesaw State University, Kennesaw, Georgia

PHYLLIS SHARPS, PhD, RN, CNE, FAAN, Professor, Department of Community-Public Health, School of Nursing, Johns Hopkins University, Baltimore, Maryland

CHARLES D. SMITH, MD, Sanders-Brown Center on Aging, Alzheimer's Disease Center; Department of Neurology and Magnetic Resonance Imaging Center, College of Medicine, University of Kentucky, Lexington, Kentucky

PATRICIA M. SPECK, DNSc, FNP-BC, FAAN, FAAFS, DF-IAFN, SANE-A, SANE-P, Assistant Professor and Public Health Nursing Option Coordinator, College of Nursing, The University of Tennessee Health Science Center, Memphis, Tennessee

MARCIA STANHOPE, RN, DSN, FAAN, Professor and Good Samaritan Endowed Chair in Community Health Nursing, College of Nursing, University of Kentucky, Lexington, Kentucky

LISA SUMMERS, CNM, MSN, DrPH, Director of Professional Services, American College of Nurse Midwives, Silver Spring, Maryland

LISA M. TURNER, MSN, APRN, BC, Research Intern, Good Samaritan Nursing Center, College of Nursing, University of Kentucky, Lexington, Kentucky

LORRI VELTEN, MBA, Director for Payor Relations, School of Medicine, Texas Tech University–Health Sciences Center, Lubbock, Texas

CECILIA M. WACHDORF, PhD, CNM, Clinical Assistant Professor, University of Minnesota School of Nursing, Minneapolis, Minnesota

YAN ZHANG, PhD, Assistant Professor, Department of Family and Community Medicine, School of Medicine, Texas Tech University–Health Sciences Center, Lubbock, Texas

CONTENTS

Health Education Through Extension Leaders (HEEL) is one of the solutions the University of Kentucky College of Agriculture has created to address the problem of chronic disease in Kentucky. Building on the land grant model for education, outreach, and prevention, HEEL collaborates and partners with the academic health centers, area health education centers, the Center for Rural Health, the Kentucky Cancer Program, the Markey Cancer Center, the University of Kansas Wellness Program, and the Kentucky Cabinet for Health and Family Services to implement research-based preventive programs to the county extension agents across Kentucky. Extension agents are an instrumental bridge between the communities across Kentucky and the educational resources provided by the HEEL program.

The Good Samaritan Nursing Center (GSNC) is an integrated nurse-managed center that serves vulnerable populations in the community. Across its 10 clinics, the GSNC helps to improve access to health care for people of all ages. The purpose of this article is to (1) describe the services and goals of the GSNC, a Commonwealth

Collaborative; (2) discuss selected outputs/outcomes from the GSNC clinics; and (3) propose recommendations for research related to the outcomes of this nurse-managed center.

Determining Standards of Care for Substance Abuse and Alcohol Use in Long-Haul Truck Drivers

Debra Gay Anderson and Peggy Riley

The trucking industry employs approximately 9 million workers, with approximately 3 million being long-haul truck drivers. Truck drivers are exposed to a variety of stressful situations, such as working long hours, no sleep, inadequate rest and relaxation, being away from home and support systems, and driving in hazardous conditions. These risk factors place the long-haul truck driver at an increased risk for possible use or abuse of alcohol and drugs. Identification of those at risk and those who are abusing alcohol and drugs is vitally important for the health of these truckers.

Promoting Oral Health Among the Inner City Homeless: A Community-Academic Partnership

Mary Lashley

Oral health care resources for the homeless are scarce, underfunded, and generally inadequate to meet the oral health needs of this population. The purpose of this program was to improve oral health among the urban homeless in a faith-based inner city mission through education, screening, and improved access to oral health care. The program provided for expanded delivery of oral health care services to the homeless while preparing students in the health professions for community-based practice with at-risk and vulnerable populations. By proactively addressing oral health needs through prevention and earlier diagnosis and treatment, morbidity, quality of life, and cost can be positively affected. Innovative, cross-disciplinary, community delivery models that involve key stakeholders at all levels are needed to address the oral health needs of the homeless and underserved adequately.

Transformation for Health: A Framework for Conceptualizing Health Behaviors in Vulnerable Populations

M. Christina Esperat, Du Feng, Yan Zhang, Yondell Masten, Seth Allcorn, Lorri Velten, Lynda Billings, Barbara Pence, and Mallory Boylan

Shedding light on the factors and circumstances that operate to bring about marginalization of groups can facilitate appropriate responses to the issue of health disparities among vulnerable groups in society. This is showing to be a seemingly intractable problem; however, it may well be that the approaches currently used to respond to the issues are not appropriate because we overlook the "realties" that really matter: those emanating from the people being visited by these circumstances themselves. Under normal conditions, human behavior can only be controlled by the individual. Facilitating an environment in which an individual can comprehend his or her internal and external realities is the first step toward transformative behavior.

This article provides two examples of approaches nursing can take to reach diverse populations of children and their families to enhance health lifestyles. First, a descriptive summary of a brief after-school intervention program aimed at influencing 8- and 9-year-old children's media habits and the prevention of negative health behaviors is presented. Design consideration for translating health lifestyles research findings into a nurse-managed inner city primary care practice is reviewed in the second example.

Pregnant women involved in violent relationships represent a population that is vulnerable for poor pregnancy and infant outcomes on several levels. This article describes the development of a "town and gown" partnership to assist pregnant women in violent relationships. Barriers and facilitating factors for research and home visitor (HV) nurse partnerships working with this vulnerable population were identified by HV participants in a qualitative focus group session. Methods used to develop and maintain the reciprocal relationship between the community (town) and academic researchers (gown) are described.

Kentucky's African-American Dementia Outreach Partnership (AADOP) has shown that African-American patients seek dementia care if a clinic is conveniently located and families are educated about the distinction between normal aging and signs of disease. The early identification of dementia allows African Americans access to pharmaceutic treatments that work best early in the course of the disease and provides the opportunity for the patient to plan future care. In the AADOP model, a conveniently located clinic and access to the patient's home were first steps in achieving equality of care. The trust that was built in the community through collaboration with African-American churches has allowed patients and their families to receive help with memory problems and to feel comfortable in seeking help for other medical problems. Maintaining this involvement and responsiveness to the community over the long term is the next challenge for the program.

Emergencies that challenge the infrastructure of the current health care system require a shift in the standard of usual practice. Pregnant women and their newborns are intimately linked special populations that require continued care despite the community circumstances. Pre-event planning with community partners can generate a safer alternative for providing care during a public health emergency. Lessons learned from international and United States public health emergencies have resulted in a better understanding of the essentials of care and the development of resources to guide planning for these populations.

One of the most vulnerable and voiceless groups of patients within American hospitals and institutions today are those who are dying. Health care institutions struggle with the challenge of providing excellent palliative and end-of-life care to patients while providing curative therapies at the same time. This article describes the efforts and accomplishments of the ethics committee of a community hospital system to provide for the palliative and end-of-life needs of its patients.

Substance abuse and addiction are chronic conditions characterized by an inability to control one's urge to use mood- or mind-altering drugs. Recognition of the association between addictions and crime to support the addiction, along with the relapsing nature of addictions, presents treatment and management challenges for clinicians and frustration for patients and their families. Pressures to reduce the burgeoning jail population have resulted in collaboration between the treatment community and the court—a diversion program called drug court. This article reviews the drug court programs, the clients, and the processes of accountability that direct the progress toward sobriety in the drug court clients. It also argues that the drug court clients have unique health needs requiring interventions best suited for the recovering addict enrolled in a diversion program within the criminal justice system. Nurses have the ability to influence these systems and provide safety-net clinics to drug court clients through outreach, case finding, and culturally and linguistically appropriate care that can ultimately help this population to reach a higher level of wellness.

FORTHCOMING ISSUES

RECENT ISSUES

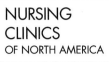

NURSING
CLINICS
OF NORTH AMERICA

ELSEVIER
SAUNDERS

Nurs Clin N Am 43 (2008) xiii–xvi

Preface

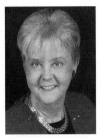

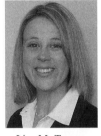

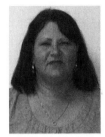

Marcia Stanhope,
RN, DSN, FAAN

Lisa M. Turner,
MSN, APRN, BC
Guest Editors

Peggy Riley, RN, MSN

In 2000, when the federal government released the document *Healthy People 2010* [1] one of the two goals for the initiative was to eliminate health disparities that occur by race and ethnicity, gender, education, income, geographic location, disability status, or sexual orientation. With the focus on improving the health of the nation through improvements in the health status of individuals, populations, and communities, one of the leading health indicators identified was access to care. The goal of eliminating disparities and the leading health indicator are intertwined because in order to eliminate health disparities, one must have access to care. The barriers to such access are noted in the document as financial, structural, and personal: lack of health insurance; low income (financial); lack of a health care provider to meet basic and special needs; lack of availability of health care facilities (structural); culture, religion, and language barriers; lack of knowledge about health care seeking behaviors; and concerns about confidentiality and discrimination (personal). When the barriers to care are compared to the population identifiers where disparities are likely to exist, it is easy to see the relationship between the goal and the health indicator and the need to improve access in order to eliminate the disparities in health status, life expectancy, and quality of life for individuals, populations, and communities.

The population identifiers above are often those that are used to describe the concept of vulnerability, or those people most likely to have little or no

doi:10.1016/j.cnur.2008.05.001

access to care and those at risk for poorer health status. Vulnerability is a global as well as a local issue, with the populations and communities who are defined as vulnerable changing depending on geographic location and the individual's, as well as the community's, level of risk for developing particular health problems [2]. Health care initiatives and partnerships targeted at access to care for the most vulnerable are essential to assisting the United States in moving toward eliminating health disparities. In the 2005 Healthy People 2010 midcourse review [3], there are mixed reviews about the health disparity objectives. Much work is needed to make a difference by 2010.

While there are many worthy goals, the 2010 objectives chosen to measure progress toward improving access to care were increased proportion of persons with health insurance (with a specific source of ongoing care) and the proportion of pregnant women who begin prenatal care in the first trimester of pregnancy. While the midcourse review did not have data on access for pregnant women, more recent data indicate that the problem of access as a result of lack of health insurance has worsened. In 2000 there were 40 million uninsured persons in the United States. In 2008 there are 47 million, or 15.6% of the total population. The numbers of uninsured children has risen slightly from 11 million to 11.7 million of all children under age 18. Similarly, in 2000, 40 million persons did not have an ongoing source of health care. This figure included both the insured and uninsured. Today, it is reported that there has been an 11% increase in the numbers of persons with an ongoing source of health care [2].

This issue of *Nursing Clinics of North America* highlights eleven projects that are assisting with improving access to care and an ongoing source of health care to vulnerable populations, some with and some without health insurance. Conceptual models are proposed and tested, application of old and new models of health care delivery are described, and interventions are used or recommended. Often, nurses work with vulnerable populations who do not have access to care, and who have or are at risk for poorer health status then the population at large. These projects emphasize the work of nurses with individuals, populations, and communities. These projects involve those who experience homelessness, who live in poverty, who are pregnant, migrant workers, immigrants, developmentally disabled, abused, victims of violence, or substance abusers. These projects also focus on particular age groups, such as children and the older adult, and particular health problems and life stages, such as chronic disease and death. Geographic locations include inner city, urban, and rural.

The article by Esperat and colleagues presents a new evidenced-based model for conceptualizing, and explaining how to predict and intervene in health behavior management with vulnerable populations. The model is applied with interventions at the individual and community level. Danner and colleagues discuss an intervention aimed at early identification of dementia in African American clients, a population the authors say may not have equal access to care and may wait longer to seek care when needed.

Involvement with the churches assists in building trust in the community. Eddy and colleagues describe a "town and gown" partnership to address the problem of pregnant women in violent relationships. Kennedy and Floriani describe their work with children and their families, aimed at enhancing healthy lifestyles through an after-school intervention program and an inner city primary care practice. Lashley focuses on the development of interprofessional and community partnerships as a way to address the oral health care needs of an urban homeless population in a faith based inner city shelter.

Education, screening, and improved access are emphasized. Pfeiffer and colleagues offer insights into lessons learned about the essentials of care and the development of resources to provide care to pregnant women and their newborn children during a public health emergency. Community partners and pre-event planning are noted as a must. Robley discusses a community hospital experience in providing palliative and end-of-life care needs for the dying patient. Speck and colleagues address the problem of the over burdened prison system and the positive results of providing a community-based drug court program of rehabilitation for persons accused of drug-related crimes. Because incarceration of the addict involved in petty crime has resulted in relapse (and often additional criminal activity) the authors argue that nurses can provide safety net clinics to assist these persons to a higher level of wellness. Anderson and Riley share the woes of the long haul truck driver, exposed to stress, long working hours, little sleep, lack of a support system, and hazardous road conditions. These risk factors, they say, expose the worker to possible use and abuse of a variety of substances. Riley further describes a statewide project aimed at improving the health status of a total population. This project involves a college of agriculture, five health care colleges, and county extension agents, as but a few of the partners in this endeavor, to address the chronic disease problem in a state that is largely rural and where more than half of the counties are in designated "medically underserved" areas.

Finally, Turner and Stanhope paint a picture of an integrated virtual nurse-managed center that provides primary and community health care services to children and adults of all ages through ten community-based sites located in schools and free clinics, including two clinics for the homeless and one for new babies and their families. A geomap shows the outreach to children in four elementary schools, and the outputs of the center are described over time. Foundation, education, health department, and university partners are highlighted.

While the projects discussed highlight the work of nurses and the impact the nursing profession can have on improving health care access, the articles also highlight the effects that community and interprofessional partnerships have on enhancing and sustaining these projects. At any given time in any location all of us may become vulnerable. A health condition for which we have been at risk may emerge. Because we are not the gatekeepers of the health care system, as individuals we may be denied access, as one author recently learned through a personal experience. As we can envision through these projects and interventions, nurses can help break the cycle of vulnerability and improve health care access for all, regardless of existing individual, population, and community circumstances.

Marcia Stanhope, RN, DSN, FAAN
Professor and Good Samaritan Endowed Chair in Community Health Nursing
College of Nursing
University of Kentucky
Lexington, Kentucky USA

E-mail address: marcia.stanhope@uky.edu

Lisa M. Turner, MSN, APRN, BC
Research Intern
Good Samaritan Nursing Center
College of Nursing
University of Kentucky
Lexington, Kentucky USA

E-mail address: lmpede3@uky.edu

Peggy Riley, RN, MSN
Extension Health Specialist for Nursing
Health Education through Extension Leadership Program
College of Agriculture and College of Nursing
University of Kentucky
Lexington, Kentucky USA

E-mail address: parile2@uky.edu

References

[1] US Department of Health and Human Services. Healthy people 2010: understanding and improving. Washington DC, US: Government Printing Office; 2001.
[2] Sebastian J. Vulnerability and vulnerable populations. In Stanhope M, Lancaster J. Public Health Nursing: Population Centered Health Care in the Community. 7th edition, 2008, Mosby, St Louis, MO.
[3] US Department of Health and Human Services. Healthy people 2010: midcourse review. Washington DC, US: Government Printing Office; 2005.

NURSING
CLINICS
OF NORTH AMERICA

Nurs Clin N Am 43 (2008) 329–340

Collaboration for Prevention of Chronic Disease in Kentucky: The Health Education Through Extension Leaders (HEEL) Program

Peggy Riley, RN, MSN

Health Education through Extension Leadership Program, College of Agriculture and College of Nursing, University of Kentucky, 10 Erikson Hall, Lexington, KY 859-257-8900, USA

Addressing the diverse health care needs of Kentuckians is a challenge. Finding ways to deliver health promotion and preventive education to communities across the state to eliminate or decrease chronic disease should be a priority. The collaborative partnership between the College of Nursing and the College of Agriculture Health Education Through Extension Leaders (HEEL) program provides the opportunity to assist in the effort to decrease or eliminate chronic disease in Kentuckians through preventive health education.

Extension health specialists, who have shared appointments between the academic health centers and the HEEL program, create health education programming, then partner with cooperative extension agents across the state to bring educational materials to the culturally diverse communities across the state.

Cooperative extension agents live and work in the communities they serve. This unique working environment provides specialists the conduit needed to deliver culturally specific health information to community members across the state. Approximately one half of Kentucky residents live in rural, isolated regions without access to health education and resources.

Living and working in the community also provides cooperative extension agents with the ability to form sustainable partnerships and coalitions to promote health within these communities. Further, cooperative extension

The development of the HEEL program was made possible by Senator Mitch McConnell with funds earmarked for the University of Kentucky, College of Agriculture, Lexington, KY and budgeted through the CSREES/USDA Federal Administration.

E-mail address: parile2@uky.edu

agents know the communities' health needs and the cultural diversity of the communities and are able to adapt programming to fit those needs.

Significance of health problems in Kentucky

The top six leading causes of death in Kentucky are heart disease, stroke, cancer, chronic obstructive pulmonary disease (Kentucky ranks fifth in the nation for deaths), unintentional injury, and diabetes (leading cause of disability) [1]. These chronic diseases have often been called the "Kentucky uglies."

Kentucky has the third highest age-adjusted rate of heart disease in the country. Heart disease is the leading cause of death in Kentucky. Directly contributing to heart disease are smoking, sedentary lifestyle, and poor nutrition [2]. Ranking for Kentucky on these key modifiable health risk behaviors is summarized in Table 1 [3]. Diabetes has been recognized as the leading cause of death and disability in Kentucky [2]. Prevention of these debilitating and often fatal chronic diseases is the primary goal of the College of Agriculture, Cooperative Extension Service, the HEEL program, and College of Nursing research program [4–6]. According to the Kentucky Behavioral Risk Factor Surveillance System [7], "one-fourth of the adult population do not participate in any type of leisure time physical activity, 32.6% of the adult population are current smokers, and 62.5% of the adult population are overweight" (Table 2). Youth risk factors are summarized in Table 3. One third of the adult population has high blood pressure and 25% have high cholesterol [7,8]. For the year 2002, Kentucky had the highest smoking prevalence in the nation and one in four adult Kentuckians are obese [7,8].

Further compounding the risk factors is that Kentucky is approximately 42.8% rural. In some areas of the state it may take hours to get to the nearest health care facility or doctor's office. This distance creates a complexity for addressing some of these major health concerns. Prevention of chronic disease and health promotion may be inaccessible to these residents.

Establishment of need for preventive health education

According to the Kentucky Institute of Medicine, Health of Kentucky Report of 2007, most chronic disease in Kentucky can be eliminated or decreased with lifestyle modifications [9]. Behavioral risk factors, such as tobacco use,

Table 1
Ranking for risk behaviors

Risk factor	Kentucky	United states	Rank
Smoking rates (adult)	28.2%	20.6%	1
Obesity rates (adults)	27.5%	24.4%	7
High blood pressure (adults)	29.4%	25%	7
Medical cost of obesity (per capita)	$282	$258	15

Data from Trust for America's health. The state of your health: Kentucky, 2006. Available at: http://healthyamericans.org/state/print.php?StateID=KY. Accessed January 3, 2008.

Table 2
Risk factors for chronic disease: percent of Kentucky adults

Risk factor	%
High cholesterol	25
Overweight/obese	63
Physical inactivity	31
Not eating recommended fruits and vegetables	78
Smoking	32.6

Data from Kentucky Behavioral Risk Factor Surveillance System. BRFSS 2002 Report. Kentucky Department for Public Health: Frankford, KY; 2004. Available at: http://chfs.ky. gov/dph/epi/brfss.htm. Accessed January 3, 2008.

poor diet, and physical inactivity, are the leading causes of mortality-linked disease, such as cardiovascular disease, cancer, and diabetes.

Several factors play a significant role in laying the foundation for the poor health status of Kentuckians: topography of the state, demographics, and access to health care. Topographically 85 of Kentucky's 120 counties are rural with one half of Kentuckians living in those rural regions. Some of these rural counties are located in remote and isolated regions of the state. In some areas of the state it may take hours to get to the nearest health care facility or doctor [9]. To these Kentuckians, prevention is a necessity to prevent development of minor health problems into chronic disease.

Demographics play another major role in the poor health status of Kentuckians. Lack of education has been linked with an increased risk

Table 3
Risk factors for chronic disease: youth

Risk factor	%
Smoking	
Male	31.8
Female	33.4
Physical inactivity	
Male	7.9
Female	13.2
Not eating recommended fruits and vegetables	
Male	86
Female	88
Overweight	
Male	19.5
Female	9.5
At risk for becoming overweight	
Male	14.4
Female	16.4
At risk for diabetes	
Male	11.8
Female	14.9

Data from Kentucky Behavioral Risk Factor Surveillance System. BRFSS 2002 Report. Kentucky Department for Public Health: Frankford, KY; 2004. Available at: http://chfs.ky. gov/dph/epi/brfss.htm. Accessed January 3, 2008.

for poor health status. People who have low educational attainment may not have access to preventive health education. Further, those who have lower education are more likely to practice poor lifestyle behaviors, such as poor nutrition, smoking, and lack of physical activity. Kentucky has one of the higher low-education rates in the nation, ranking 48th out of 50. Those who have lower education may also end up in low-paying jobs that do not offer health insurance [9].

Poverty is another factor contributing to poor health. Kentucky has the eighth highest poverty rate in the United States and is fourth highest for the number of older people living in poverty. According to the Kentucky Institute of Medicine, "Kentucky has 43 high-poverty counties, with poverty rates of 20% or higher, and 35 of the poorest counties in terms of the latest estimates by the U.S. Bureau of Economic Analysis." Thirty-three of those Kentucky counties have been classified by the Appalachian Regional Commission. Barriers these Kentuckians must face include low-paying jobs without health insurance and poor living standards, which may lead to increased risk for low health status [9].

Lack of health access is another contributing factor to the health status of Kentuckians. According to recent estimates half a million Kentuckians are uninsured, with the highest percentage being children and young adults aged 18 to 25. County uninsured rates range from 8% to 25%. According to the Kentucky Institute of Medicine, Health of Kentucky 2007 report, "in 2004, the lack of health insurance was the cause of 18,000 unnecessary deaths per year in the U.S." Although strides have been made across the United States and in Kentucky for employers to provide health insurance, problems may arise because of existing medical conditions and existing poor health status causing insurance costs to be higher or not available. The uninsured are also less likely to seek preventive health care, fill needed prescriptions, and get care for acute illness that can lead to complications or chronic disease [9].

A decreased primary care physician/population ratio also creates a problem. The ratio for Kentucky is 2.5 per 3500 compared with the United States at 3.7 per 3500. Having access to a primary care physician increases the likelihood of seeking preventive health care [9].

Background of health education through extension leaders program

A brief history of the land grant model and emergence of extension is provided in this section. It is impossible to discuss the importance of the collaboration between the College of Nursing and the College of Agriculture HEEL program, or the development of the HEEL program, without providing the framework on which this program was established. The HEEL program has its roots in three entities: the land grant system, the Cooperative Extension Service, and University of Kentucky Academic Health Centers [10].

The land grant system provides the basic foundation for the HEEL program. The land grant system, created by the Morrill Act of 1862, provided public lands for establishment of colleges for the benefit of agriculture, home economics, and mechanical arts. Building on this foundation is the Cooperative Extension Service. The Cooperative Extension Service was created by the Smith-Lever Act of 1914. This act allowed local governments to become legal partners with the State and Federal Government to bring the research from the land-grant universities to the people at the local level. A formal partnership between the land grant colleges and the United States Department of Agriculture (USDA) was formed with this act [11]. The gap between the people of the Commonwealth of Kentucky and the land grant institutions was bridged with this act, hence bringing university expertise to the people of the state. Education and research filtered down to local communities giving them access to resources they may never have had [12]. Extension agents bring leadership, community education, and organizational skills to the table. Agents work to form community partnerships and engage expertise from the universities to assist communities in identifying and taking appropriate action to problem solve [12–14]. The importance of these skills is essential in the HEEL program collaboration between the extension health specialists and the cooperative extension agents. Agents assist the extension health specialists in identifying community leaders and key personnel for formation of coalitions and other partnerships to promote health.

Enhancement of the Cooperative Extension Service was made possible by the creation of the Cooperative State Research, Education, and Extension Service (CSREES). Creation of CSREES was accomplished by the Department Reorganization Act of 1994. This branch of federal government is housed within the USDA. The act combined the USDA's Cooperative State Research Service and the Extension Service to bring together expertise in research, education, and extension, creating streamlined leadership to enhance outreach of these agencies [11].

Dissemination of knowledge is at the heart of this agency's mission. Knowledge dissemination is accomplished through state, regional, and county extension offices. Agents from these offices respond to community needs and requests and provide educational events and workshops based on these needs. Materials provided by this network are grounded in evidence-based research made possible by the land grant institutions. Extension means reaching out. Along with teaching and research, land grant institutions extend their resources, solving public needs with college or university resources [11].

The Kentucky Cooperative Extension Service is the result of a unique cooperative agreement between the University of Kentucky, Kentucky State University, the USDA, and each Kentucky County. It provides lifelong, continuing education for the people of the Commonwealth. Extension's strength is the involvement of people in the process of planning, developing, and performing programs that meet their needs. Since the beginning of extension, it has been assumed that people must be reached where they are in their level of understanding. Extension's focus on people is through programs in which self-improvement is encouraged. The primary focus of the Kentucky Cooperative Extension Service is to assist people to identify problems and their solutions through the delivery of new knowledge and assistance in its implementation. To accomplish this, extension arranges for significant involvement of the public in planning and conducting programs, thereby transferring relevant technology and information to the general public [4,15].

The Kentucky Cooperative Extension Service is the educational resource that serves as a catalyst to build better communities and improve quality of life for all Kentuckians. Further, the Cooperative Extension Service serves as the link between the counties of the Commonwealth and the state's land grant universities to help people improve their lives through an educational process focusing on their issues and needs [4,15].

Another key factor in the establishment of the HEEL program is the accessibility of expertise made available through the university's Academic Health Centers. The Academic Health Centers consist of the Colleges of Dentistry, Medicine, Nursing, Pharmacy, and Public Health. The University of Kentucky is one of a few land grant universities that house all seven of the Academic Health Centers on one campus [10]. Having expertise and research abilities on one campus greatly enhances sustainability of the HEEL program. In addition, the College of Public Health houses the National Institute of Occupational Safety and Health–funded Southeast Center for Agricultural Health and Injury Prevention. This center is directed by the Department of Preventive Medicine and the Environmental Health in College of Public Health and the College of Agriculture, with main emphasis on issues affecting agricultural families, such as aging farmers, tractor safety, and other health-related issues specific to agriculture [10,16].

Initial program planning for HEEL involved a state health needs assessment to identify Kentucky-specific health promotion and preventive education needs. This assessment, along with need for agent enhancement of community health education needs, was presented to University and Academic Health Center College administration. As noted by HEEL program founders, agents were already doing health education on topics such as cancer prevention and nutrition, but there was weakness because the programs were based on the agent's knowledge, not on evidence-based practice [10,12,16,17]. Framework for the HEEL project is centered on bridging the infrastructure of the College of Medicine's School of Public Health with the College of Agriculture's Cooperative Extension Service based on goals from Healthy People 2010 and Healthy Kentuckians 2010, creating a blueprint for increasing the quality and availability of community-based educational programs addressing prevention, mortality rates, and promotion of health and well-being in Kentucky [5,10]. Funding for the HEEL program is made possible from funds earmarked from Senator Mitch McConnell to the USDA and CSREES [5].

The goal of HEEL is based on HP 2010 Objective 7 for educational and community-based programs, with the goal of increasing the quality and effectiveness of educational and community-based programs designed to prevent disease and improve health and quality of life. HEEL serves as a catalyst for change by bridging people, resources, ideas, and actions, using the unique land grant model of outreach and education combined with university-based research and formal collaborations with long-term partnerships [5].

Initial HEEL campus collaborative partnerships were with the College of Dentistry, College of Medicine, College of Public Health, College of Pharmacy, and the College of Social Work. Social work was added to program needs to enhance mental health issues that can have negative health impacts. In 2005, HEEL partnered with the College of Nursing to bring expertise from the nursing profession, specifically public health nursing. Through the years, collaborative partnerships have also been formed with the area health education centers, the Center for Rural Health, the Kentucky Cancer Program, the Markey Cancer Center, the University of Kentucky Wellness Program, Kentucky State University, the Kentucky Diabetes Network, and the Kentucky Cabinet for Health and Family Services. In more recent years, HEEL has formed partnerships with out-of-state extension agents and other Kentucky universities to broaden the knowledge and research expertise, further enhancing delivery of health promotion and preventive health education to the state [5].

The programming objectives include education and empowerment of individuals and families to adopt healthy behaviors and lifestyles, build community capacity to improve health, and educate consumers to make informed health choices. Programming created by HEEL is to be delivered by cooperative extension agents. Extension agents come from various backgrounds but all have expertise in delivering community education. To further enhance program delivery, agents are instrumental in developing local coalitions to examine and become involved in prevention of chronic disease. The extension health specialists representing collaborating colleges and partnerships serve as the bridge between the HEEL program and the respective colleges' research. Extension health specialists disseminate research and help place cutting-edge information into practice. Materials for HEEL programs have undergone extensive examination and review by professionals in the medical community and the social science community and peer collaborators who have expertise in various fields [5].

Programming is based on the train-the-trainer model for education. Train-the-trainer models have been used by various audiences from business to health care. Because of the many job responsibilities, agents sometimes must rely on program assistants and other volunteers to assist with program delivery. Using a train-the-trainer model for delivering HEEL programming allows the extension specialist to become the program manager, ensuring the program is delivered as it should be and evaluations are completed, and ensuring accurate data are collected about program impact. The train-the-trainer model also increases the knowledge base of the agent and program assistants and volunteers. Program participants feel more at ease and are more inclined to participate in the program if it is given by peers or those who have similar cultural and socioeconomic backgrounds [18–20].

Target audiences for HEEL educational resources are rural and urban limited resource audiences, communities with limited resources, farm operators, agricultural and forestry workers and their families, health volunteers and professionals, infants, children, young adults, seniors, and special populations, such as high-risk teens and families. Educational resources address topics such as childhood obesity, adult physical activity and obesity, cancer, injury prevention, cardiovascular disease, substance abuse, mental health, aging, and diabetes [5].

Merging nursing and extension

Nursing and extension professionals share several qualities. Nursing strives to meet the health care needs of individuals, families, and communities across the life span using a holistic approach. Nursing takes into consideration the diversity of individuals, families, and communities, each with uniqueness and specific cultural needs. Nursing, like extension, serves all individuals regardless of race, sex, or national origin. Each also recognizes that learning is a lifelong process, with specific learning needs at each level of life.

The extension process is not unlike the nursing process: assessment, diagnosis, intervention, and evaluation [4].

Assessment: Periodically agents undergo program planning for the next 4 years. A situation analysis is conducted in each community to assess situations and issues influencing the lives of the people there.

Diagnosis: Community members are involved in assisting agents to identify specific needs. During this phase the agent forms collaborative community partnerships to further assist with identifying community needs and available community resources. Target audiences are determined along with a needs assessment of the target audience.

Intervention: Program objectives are set and content and learning strategies for the target audience are determined. The logic model is used to guide the agent through the program planning process.

Evaluation: program evaluations are built into programming materials. Participants are generally given a pretest, posttest, and overall program evaluation. In addition, agents gather information called impact statements, which directly reflect knowledge gained by program participants. An annual report is made to community members showing the impact programming has made in their specific community.

Role of the extension health specialist for nursing

The extension health specialist for nursing at the University of Kentucky is one of the first in the nation. The specialist shares a position between the College of Nursing and the HEEL program, bringing expertise and evidence-based resources from the College of Nursing. Programming focus for the specialist is chronic disease. Responsibilities include managing the Literacy, Eating, and Activity for Preschoolers (LEAP) program, which addresses childhood obesity. The target audience is children aged 3 to 5 years. The program consists of a series of 10 storybooks that teach children about making healthy food choices (more fruits and vegetables) and encouraging the children to eat more nutritious meals and increasing physical activity. Each lesson has a parent newsletter that contains information about making healthy eating choices and a recipe the parents and child/children can make together. In addition, the program has a lesson about oral health that teaches preschoolers the importance of taking care of their teeth and gums for prevention of disease. The program is taught in preschools, daycare centers, Head Start programs, and other sites, such as churches, schools, and community centers. The program is currently undergoing expansion to include early elementary–aged children.

Additional programming addresses health issues, such as diabetes, cancer prevention, cardiovascular disease, injury prevention, osteoporosis, and arthritis.

Monthly health bulletins are created by the specialist for adults and youth about chronic disease prevention. These bulletins are used by the extension agents. Issues are addressed, such as cancer, smoking, heart disease, injury prevention, seasonal flu, handwashing to decrease the spread of germs, and sun safety, and currently arising issues, such as methicillin-resistant *Staphylococcus aureus*, and lead poisoning. The youth bulletin compliments the adult bulletin by addressing similar topics. In addition, six youth bulletins, for middle and high school students, focus on careers in health care.

The specialist also takes part in consumer radio announcements in partnership with Agricultural Communications. These are 1-minute radio announcements addressing health issues facing Kentuckians. Half-hour radio segments are also done in partnership with a local Spanish radio station addressing health issues of migrant farm workers and the Hispanic population.

The specialist also assists extension agents with health fairs. Agents conduct health fairs throughout the year addressing various health issues. The specialist assists the agent with displays, demonstrations, and presentations at these health fairs. Another programming focus for the specialist is extension homemaker lessons. Extension homemakers are generally older, retired community members. Lessons specific to the aging population or those who have disability are designed.

One of the newest programs initiated by the specialist to enhance the work of extension agents across the state is the Master Health Education

Volunteer Program. This program is based on other Extension Master programs in which training is provided to community volunteers who wish to learn more about a topic. In exchange for learning this new material, volunteers sign a contract saying they will "pay back" their training time by going into the community to teach others. Lesson materials for the program are derived from current HEEL programming.

Information releases, fact sheets, and health alerts are also prepared by the specialist. These resources are used by agents across the state for health education. The specialist also serves as the major resource person for the agents. Health displays, video tapes, DVDs, pamphlets, and other educational materials are managed by the specialist as agent resource materials. The specialist also assists the agent in finding appropriate resources regarding emerging health issues of concern to their communities.

Advocacy is another major role for the specialist. The specialist serves on several advisory committees at the state level addressing topics such as osteoporosis, arthritis, cancer, diabetes, and obesity. The specialist advocates the importance of extension in delivering health education materials to their communities and assisting the agent to partner with these agencies.

Impact of health education and promotion on Kentuckians

Some highlights of chronic disease programming conducted last year include childhood obesity, diabetes, cancer prevention, and chronic disease prevention.

Childhood obesity

In 2007, 10,731 children aged 3 to 5 years participated in the LEAP program. Of those participating 77% reported a knowledge increase about nutrition and physical activity, 74% reported an increase in daily consumption of fruits and vegetables, 90% immediately demonstrated an increase in physical activity, 65% began a regular physical activity program, and 100% of parents reported a change in how they planned meals.

Diabetes

A presentation, entitled "Diabetes and Physical Activity," was given to a group of 150 participants in the annual Diabetes Health Expo in Mason County. This presentation was in partnership with the Mason County Family Consumer Science (FCS) agent and the District Health Department. The presentation included materials on understanding diabetes and the importance of daily physical activity and diabetes. Of those participating in the program, 100% stated they increased their knowledge of diabetes and 90% stated they would begin a daily physical activity program.

Cancer prevention

A display on sun safety, a DermaScan, and fact sheets were provided for a health fair in Bourbon County. This fair was a partnership between the Bourbon County FCS Agent, Program Assistant, local emergency medical service, and the local health department. Approximately 500 participants attended the health fair. Participants used the DermaScan to identify sun damage to their face, were given fact sheets about protecting the skin, and were engaged in a question/answer session on sun safety. Of those participating in the program, 100% were able to recognize sun damage to their faces and 80% said they would practice some type of sun safety.

Chronic disease prevention

A presentation was given to 150 participants at the annual conference for independent living, entitled "Staying Healthy to Prevent Chronic Disease." This presentation was a partnership between the Shelby County Family and Consumer Science Extension Agent and the State Disability/Handicapped Division. The presentation discussed statistics on chronic disease, impact of chronic disease, physical activity, proper nutrition, questions you should ask your doctor, importance of a family medical history, know your numbers, and importance of regular health check-ups and screenings. A demonstration on content of fats and sugars in food, food labeling, and nutritional content of food was given by the agent. Of the those participating in the presentation, 100% reported an increase in knowledge about chronic disease and how to prevent it, 100% reported an increase in knowledge of reading food labels and nutritional content of food, and 95% reported they would incorporate the staying healthy tips into their daily life.

Summary

Kentucky's health care needs are diverse and culturally different. The number of Kentuckians at risk for chronic disease or who have chronic disease greatly outnumbers the number of qualified health care professionals available to conduct preventive and promotional health education. It is vital, therefore, to engage in collaborative partnerships with professionals who possess knowledge about community education, leadership, and culture to enhance health care professionals' efforts to eliminate or decrease chronic disease.

The collaboration between the College of Nursing and the HEEL program is a sustainable partnership. Nursing and extension have numerous practice similarities, such as cultural awareness and holistic care. Working in partnership will promote health education across Kentucky to eliminate or decrease chronic disease in Kentuckians. Because extension agents live and work in the communities they are quickly able to identify emerging health care needs of the people they serve and relay that information to the extension health specialist for nursing.

References

[1] Centers for Disease Control and Prevention. Chronic diseases: the leading causes of death. Kentucky: U.S. Department of Health and Human Services, Centers for Disease Control and Prevention, National Center for Chronic Disease Prevention and Health Promotion; 2006.

[2] Health status of Kentuckians 1999. Available at: http://chfs.ky.gov/NR/rdonlyres/09215B6F-2D8C-4288-8073-A93B3483CCCE/0/healthstatusofkentuckians.pdf. Accessed December 21, 2007.

[3] Trust for America's health. The state of your health: Kentucky, 2006. Available at: http://healthyamericans.org/state/print.php?StateID=KY. Accessed December 21, 2007.

[4] University of Kentucky Cooperative Extension. History, mission, vision. Available at: http://ces.ca.uky.edu/ces/ABOUTCES.HTM. Accessed December 21, 2007.

[5] Health Education through Extension Leadership (HEEL). Program development, 2005. Available at: http://www.ca.uky.edu/heel. Accessed December 21, 2007.

[6] University of Kentucky, College of Nursing. Mission, vision statement, 2007. Available at: http://www.mc.uky.edu/Nursing/intro/phil.htm. Accessed December 22, 2007.

[7] Kentucky BRFSS. 2002. Available at: http://chfs.ky.gov/dph/epi/brfss.htm. Accessed December 22, 2007.

[8] Close to the heart of Kentucky, 2004: a report on the status of cardiovascular disease in the Commonwealth. Available at: http://chfs.ky.gov/NR/rdonlyres/BD7C096B-C412-44A8-A21E-FE061BC5EFBB/012004cvdburdenreport.pdf. Accessed December 22, 2007.

[9] Kentucky institute of medicine: the health of Kentucky: a county assessment, Lexington, Kentucky, 2007. Available at: http://kyiom.org/healthyky2007a.pdf. Accessed December 21, 2007.

[10] Scutchfield DF, Harris TT, Tanner B, et al. Academic health centers and cooperative extension service: a model for a working partnership. Journal of Extension 2007;45(1). Available at: www.joe.org. Accessed December 21, 2007.

[11] United States Department of Agriculture, CSREES. CSREES overview. Journal of Extension 2007;45:1. Article number 1FEA5.

[12] Griner-Hill L, Parker LA. Extension as a delivery system for prevention programming: capacity, barriers, and opportunities. Journal of Extension 2005;(1):43. Article number 1FEA1. Available at: www.joe.org. Accessed January 5, 2008.

[13] Peters S. Rousing the people on the land: the roots of the educational organizing tradition in extension work. Journal of Extension 2002;40(3). Available at: www.joe.org. Accessed January 5, 2008.

[14] Fehlis CP. A call for visonary leadership. Journal of Extension 2002;40(3). Available at: www.joe.org. Accessed January 5, 2008.

[15] University of Kentucky extension manual: a reference on policies and procedures for extension agents, University of Kentucky cooperative extension service, College of Agriculture, 2000.

[16] Association of Academic Health Centers. About AAHC. 2007. Available at: www.aahdc.org. Accessed January 10, 2008.

[17] Franz N, Peterson R, Dailey A. Leading organizational change: a comparison of county and campus views of extension engagement. Journal of Extension 2005;40(3). Available at: www.joe.org. Accessed January 10, 2008.

[18] Assemi M, Mutha S, Suchanek H. Evaluation of a train-the-trainer program for cultural competence. American Association of Colleges of Pharmacy. 2006. Available at: www.aacp.org. Accessed January 10, 2008.

[19] Green ML. A train-the-trainer model for integrating evidence-based medicine training into podiatric medical education. J Am Podiatr Med Assoc 2005;95(5):496–504.

[20] Williamson C, McGlaun J, Office of Rural Health Policy. Preserving local healthcare: case studies of rural health works implementation in three communities. July 2004. Available at: http://ruralhealth.hrsa.gov/pub/RHWreport.htm. Accessed January 5, 2008.

ELSEVIER
SAUNDERS

Nurs Clin N Am 43 (2008) 341–356

NURSING
CLINICS
OF NORTH AMERICA

The Good Samaritan Nursing Center: A Commonwealth Collaborative

Lisa M. Turner, MSN, APRN, BC*,
Marcia Stanhope, RN, DSN, FAAN

*Good Samaritan Nursing Center, College of Nursing, University of Kentucky,
315 CON Building, Lexington, KY 40536-0232, USA*

Improving access to health care, reducing health disparities, and promoting the health of vulnerable populations are all important issues integral to improving the quality of life of Americans. The Good Samaritan Nursing Center (GSNC) is an integrated nurse-managed center that addresses each of these concerns. Across its 10 clinics, the GSNC provides primary and preventive care to clients of all ages. This Center is improving health care access for those populations who would otherwise fall through the gaps. In addition to providing services for vulnerable populations, the Center works to increase the number of nurses working in public health through its internship and fellowship programs for newly graduated registered nurses (RNs) (BSN prepared) and nurse practitioners, respectively. The purpose of this article is to (1) describe the services and goals of the GSNC, a Commonwealth Collaborative, (2) discuss selected outputs/outcomes from the GSNC clinics, and (3) propose recommendations for research related to the outputs/outcomes of this nurse-managed center.

Access to health care

Improving access to health care services is needed to improve the health of Americans and to eliminate health disparities. Barriers to accessing health care include not having health insurance or lack of adequate coverage, lack of health care professions or lack of health care facilities, and personal barriers, such as a language barrier or lack of knowledge of when and

---

This work was supported by grants from the Good Samaritan Foundation, a ministry of the Kentucky Annual Conference of the United Methodist Church, Crestwood, Kentucky.

* Corresponding author.
E-mail address: lmpede3@uky.edu (L.M. Turner).

how to seek care [1]. Of these barriers, health insurance coverage is perhaps the most critical indicator of determining access to health care. Currently, there are 47 million Americans, 12.8 million of whom are children, living without health insurance [2]. People who live without health insurance are at risk for poorer health because of their lack of coverage [3]. In 2004 it was reported that roughly 18,000 unnecessary deaths occur every year in the United States because of lack of health insurance [4].

Nurse-managed centers

Nurse-managed centers are helping to reduce health disparities and improve access to health care. In addition, it has been determined through various surveys that when located in schools and colleges of nursing, these centers support the tripartite mission of colleges and universities by providing educational sites for students, practice sites and community service opportunities for faculty, and research opportunities [5–7].

Nurse-managed centers are health centers that are managed and staffed by advanced-practice or baccalaureate-prepared nurses. Nurse-managed centers are dynamic and are represented by different models of nursing and health care delivery. There are more than 200 nurse-managed centers in the United States [8]. In a survey developed and conducted by Dr. Juliann Sebastian, Dean, University of Missouri, St. Louis, and colleagues in 2003 [9], by way of contract with the Michigan Academic Consortium, several models of nurse-managed centers were described: a primary care model, a community health promotion model, a mixed model of primary care and community health promotion, and other models serving specific target populations, such as people who have diabetes and industrial workers, to name a few. These centers primarily provide care to the uninsured and underinsured, with the goal of reducing emergency room use and hospitalization among clients [10]. Nurse-managed centers essentially provide health care where health disparities are most acute: poor rural and urban communities [11]. For those who focus on vulnerable populations, nurse-managed centers meet the Institutes of Medicine definition of safety net providers [12]. The main characteristics of safety net providers are that they offer care to patients regardless of their ability to pay for those services and a considerable portion of their patient mix is uninsured, Medicaid, or other vulnerable patients [12].

Commonwealth collaborative

In the summer of 2005, the University of Kentucky identified 23 community outreach projects within the University whose purpose was to address a social, economic, or health issue, which if resolved would improve the quality of life of Kentuckians. These projects are called the Commonwealth Collaborative. The Commonwealth Collaborative project emphasizes the importance of translating research into practice so that the health of the community can be improved. This project also stresses the importance of collaborating with the community to make the translation of research into practice most successful [13].

All of the colleges across the University of Kentucky's campus were invited to submit project proposals. Only the top 23 projects that best fit with the university's community engagement goals were selected by the panel to be a Commonwealth Collaborative. The GSNC was named as one of these 23 projects. The GSNC not only addresses the project's goal of improving access to health care but it also uses community partnerships to implement goals. Community partnerships have been vital to the success of the Center. It is only with the support and encouragement from the Good Samaritan Foundation, Lexington-Fayette County Health Department, the Fayette County school system, and community health providers that the Center has been able to meet its goals.

The Good Samaritan Nursing Center: history and overview

Although the precursor to the GSNC began in 1994, the Center was formally organized within the College of Nursing in 1998. The Center established a community-based nursing practice arrangement to provide access to primary health care to unserved/underserved populations in Lexington, Kentucky and surrounding communities while expanding the education of nurses for community-oriented primary health care delivery. The Center concept was developed following the success of two programs within the College of Nursing and partially funded by the Good Samaritan Foundation. The first program established in 1994 allowed the College of Nursing to implement a community health nurse internship. This program was designed to assist new baccalaureate graduates in gaining experience and further education as community health nurses. Community-based and public health agencies, including school systems, prefer to hire graduates who can demonstrate their ability to be effective, capable providers. The nurse internship program meets this requirement by giving the baccalaureate nurse the opportunity to experience the community health nurse role. As a result of the success of the internship program the primary care nurse practitioner fellowship program was established in 1997 at the recommendation of the Foundation Board. This program provides newly graduated nurse practitioners the opportunity to mature in their role as primary care providers. The Center continues to provide internships and fellowships for newly graduated RNs (BSN prepared) who are interested in public health nursing and to nurse practitioners. According to the most recent national data available, only 15% of all nurses currently work in community/public health [14]. The Center aims to increase the numbers of community/public health nurses by mentoring new graduates and teaching them the skills they need to work in public health.

Through the GSNC the College of Nursing is able to provide access and serve the health care needs of vulnerable populations and support the programs of other community-based agencies as they provide service to populations otherwise unserved. The GSNC provides a seamless experience for the clients, which helps to reduce service fragmentation and decreases difficulty accessing a wide range of services while promoting continuity of care for clients who are mobile. The clients of the GSNC are experiencing health promotion and prevention of illness as clinical integration, over time, ensures comprehensive and uninterrupted care that is responsive to client and family concerns. The Center focuses on prevention of illness and disability and the promotion of health and optimal functional status.

The Center provides services through three primary care clinics serving children, adults, and families; four elementary school–based clinics; one middle school clinic; and two clinics that serve the homeless and people who have substance abuse problems. Clinics are strategically placed where low-income populations can be served.

Goals of the Good Samaritan Nursing Center

The goals of the Center include: (1) meeting the primary health care needs of vulnerable populations, otherwise unserved, (2) modeling best nursing practices in the community, (3) promoting comprehensive school health education to enhance the population's health, (4) establishing community partnerships, (5) promoting new graduates' development, initiative, self-reliance, and leadership in community health and primary care practice, and (6) establishing a network of community resources for meeting the population's health needs. These goals are being met through the 10 primary care clinics, a health education curriculum, and the internship/fellowship program.

The Good Samaritan Nursing Center primary health care services

The Center provides primary health care services through five community-based clinics and school health services in five schools. These services are direct care services solely operated by the GSNC or, in three of the community-based clinics, support staff is supplied by the GSNC to assist those clinics in meeting their mission. The clinics provide primary care, preventive care, acute health care, chronic health care, episodic health care, and urgent health care. Specific services have included: (1) individual and family health and cultural assessment, (2) care coordination to prevent fragmentation of services, (3) interventions with acute episodic, chronic, emergent, and urgent health problems and management, (4) ongoing assessment, monitoring, and evaluation of health problems, (5) select home visits to follow up and evaluate health problems addressed through the primary care services, (6) evaluation (for prenatal care) and assistance in obtaining specialty care and managing a healthy pregnancy, (7) age-appropriate health screening, (8) assessment of functional status, (9) medication monitoring/compliance, (10) diagnostic screening for physical and mental health, (11) immunizations, (12) health education and counseling, (13) anticipatory guidance/well child care, (14) tuberculosis therapy, and (15) follow-up care for referrals. The Center has provided more than 10,000 primary care visits per year plus more than 20,000 health promotion encounters per year. It has served more than 40,000 clients in a 10-year period.

The Good Samaritan Nursing Center community health services

In addition to the primary care services, the Center has provided community health services aimed at promoting health and preventing disease. GSNC interns developed a comprehensive health education curriculum ("ABCs of Health Education") for children in all grade levels. The interns have implemented the curriculum by developing and teaching lessons to the children in the four elementary schools in which the Center has clinics. Interns have also developed a series of interactive CD-ROM lessons that teach children the importance of helmet safety, substance use prevention, hand washing, nutrition, and exercise. Health education and promotion events have also been conducted through several health fairs offered to all schools in seven Kentucky counties. Themes of the health fairs have been safety tips, healthy body systems, and control of emotions. Other community health services offered by the center have included: (1) continuing school needs assessments, (2) population-based health risk appraisal, (3) targeted disease prevention/health promotion activities for the school populations, (4) select home visits to assess family needs, (5) health screenings, (6) community resource referrals for health, social, and economic needs that cannot be addressed by this project, (7) pregnancy prevention/family planning programming, (8) parenting skills assessment and interventions, (9) assessment of environmental hazards, (10) cultural assessment of the population, (11) case finding, and (12) mental health assessments.

The Good Samaritan Nursing Center populations served

The GSNC sees clients across the age spectrum (birth through 95 years). Most of the clients seen in the 2006–07 year were female (61%). Most clients were white (62%), followed by African American (23%), Hispanic (13%), and other (2%) [15]. These data reflect similar data found in national surveys previously mentioned. Clients served through the GSNC usually have no other known means of health care or health insurance. If a client has insurance or a community-based health provider, they are provided urgent or emergent care services and referred to their primary provider. The GSNC helps to improve access to health care by placing clinics where low-income populations can be served and provides services at no cost to the clients.

Evaluation of the center: the model

The cybernetic model of Veney and Kaluzny [16] is used as the model for planning and evaluation for the GSNC (Fig. 1). The model is supported by a definition of evaluation "as the collection and analysis of information by various methods to determine the relevance, adequacy, progress, efficiency, effectiveness, impact, and sustainability of a set of program activities" [16]. The process of planning, implementation, and evaluation is ongoing in the Center and a few select evaluative activities to date are highlighted. Numerous changes have occurred over the 10 years of the Center's existence as a result of the annual evaluation efforts.

Veney and Kaluzny [16] describe the evaluation model as a continuous series of feedback loops with the three interconnected activities of planning, implementation, and control. These three variables serve to provide evaluative information to show the status of the organization/system/program/project to be used (the Center) to continually move closer to the attainment of the goals and objectives.

Planning: relevance

In this model evaluation begins with planning and designing a project. The relevance is often established through a needs assessment to determine the project parameters. Numerous needs assessments have been conducted first to determine whether the GSNC was a feasible project, and second, to look at whether it should continue as designed and how it should change to remain relevant to the goals. The continuing assessment of relevance,

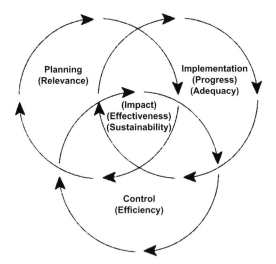

Fig. 1. Cybernetic model of program planning, implementation, and evaluation. (*From* Veney JE, Kaluzny AD. Evaluation and decision making for health services. Washington, DC: Beardbooks; 2004; with permission.)

Veney and Kaluzny [16] say, is to evaluate the impact the project is having as designed. The most recent assessment of relevance occurred through a school health task force of the local Board of Health, which involved members of the community in discussions about how to achieve the Healthy 2010 goal of a nurse in the schools for every 750 children [1]. This assessment of relevance has resulted in a new partnership arrangement between the University of Kentucky College of Nursing and the local health department to continue the work of the GSNC in the four elementary schools and one middle school as the partners work together to provide a mechanism for sustainability for the school health nurse program and the meeting of the 2010 goal. In addition, an assessment of the community needs to provide for vulnerable populations not currently served is being conducted through the local health department and community partners, including the GSNC. The culmination of this process will determine the continued role of the Center in working with the five agencies that are providing care through free clinics for those who otherwise cannot access the health care system.

Implementation: progress and adequacy

For implementation, the adequacy of the Center to address the entire problem of access to care for those unserved through schools and free clinics in a meaningful way is an important question to answer. The Center project began as a pilot to interest new baccalaureate graduates and new nurse practitioner graduates in serving vulnerable populations and developing a commitment to access to care for all regardless of circumstances. It is clear that this project in and of itself will not meet the needs of the unserved alone. It has served to substantially increase the interest of the new graduates in serving the vulnerable populations, however. The pilot has also increased the interest of other community agencies in embracing the Center as a partner in finding solutions to local needs of select populations.

Progress of the Center in conducting identified activities within budget is evaluated daily through monitoring staff activities, monthly through staff meetings, and reporting by staff of activities, encounters, and resource needs. Progress is reported every year through an annual report to the Good Samaritan Foundation that includes how well the project was conducted within the budgeted funds. Several educational issues have been addressed with staff to improve use of acceptable and professional practices; for example, discussions have been held with experts to assist staff in appropriate assessment and reporting of suspected client abuse. Emphasis is also placed on providing the new graduates with additional techniques to be used in working with clients. A process is currently in place to have all baccalaureate-prepared nurse staff trained in Early and Periodic Screening, Diagnostic, and Treatment (EPSTD) assessments to help children and families monitor the growth, development, and risk factors for the children in the schools served by the Center.

Control: efficiency

The control variable in the evaluation model refers to the efficiency of the project inputs to attain the desired outputs or outcomes. A distinction is made in the model about the use of the terms outputs and outcomes. Veney and Kaluzny [16] describe outputs as the more immediate effects of the project activities, whereas outcomes are the more long-term effects of the project activities.

Cost analyses assist in evaluating the efficiencies of a project such as the GSNC. More sophisticated analyses would include cost-benefit, cost-effectiveness, or cost-utility analyses. At this point a simple cost analysis (or checkbook analysis) has been completed to determine the cost of the GSNC activities (inputs) to the desired outputs (numbers of services offered, numbers of clients served). This simple cost analysis was performed, taking into account the cost of personnel, supplies, and equipment. Through this analysis, it was found that the services provided by the Center are done so through extremely reasonable costs. Over a 7-year period used for the analysis, the Center served a total of 40,268 individuals. For all services provided the cost was found to be $18 per individual per year. Furthermore, over the 7 years, there were 41,300 clinic visits, costing $12 per visit per year. Finally there were 127,000 health education contacts, costing $4 per contact per year. Indirect and contributed costs and resources, such as space, were not included in this analysis. The next step is a cost-benefit or cost-effectiveness analysis.

Additional efficiency analyses of services offered in the four elementary schools were conducted using the technique of trend analysis. The question addressed in these analyses was whether the presence of the GSNC and services offered accounted for changes in school attendance over time and changes in elementary students' knowledge and state-level test scores in the areas of healthy living.

Having a nursing clinic on school grounds was believed to be likely to improve attendance rates. The attendance rates were therefore reviewed for the four elementary schools and the one middle school with GSNC clinics. A paired-samples *t* test was used to test for differences between attendance rates at the school before and after establishing a clinic. Although the *t* test was not statistically significant, the attendance rate is moving in the right direction. Fig. 2 illustrates the attendance rate trends at the five GSNC schools. Furthermore, in the 2004–05 school year, all five schools had a higher attendance rate than the school district and four of the five schools had attendance rates higher than the state average.

To assess the impact of the health education taught by the baccalaureate-prepared RNs at the elementary schools, the results of the Centers for Disease Control Youth Risk Behavior Survey (YRBS) [17] and the Kentucky Core Content Tests were reviewed. The YRBS asks students about risky behaviors in various health areas, including car and play safety

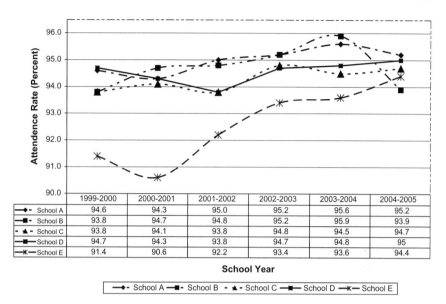

	1999-2000	2000-2001	2001-2002	2002-2003	2003-2004	2004-2005
School A	94.6	94.3	95.0	95.2	95.6	95.2
School B	93.8	94.7	94.8	95.2	95.9	93.9
School C	93.8	94.1	93.8	94.8	94.5	94.7
School D	94.7	94.3	93.8	94.7	94.8	95
School E	91.4	90.6	92.2	93.4	93.6	94.4

School Year

—◆- School A —■- School B · ▲· School C —■— School D —✳— School E

Fig. 2. Attendance rate trends at GSNC schools.

(such as seat belt use and helmet use when riding bicycles), alcohol and illegal drug use, gun and knife use, fighting, home safety (such as smoke alarms), being home alone, child and family nutrition and foods they eat/ like, exercise, use of tobacco, weight, illnesses, health care, and feelings of being happy or sad. The survey is administered by the RN interns to students with parental consent. The survey is given at the beginning of the school year and then again to the same students at the end of the school year. Survey results indicated that students at all four elementary schools showed improvement from baseline in several areas of health behaviors. Nutrition, exercise, safety, anger management, and body image were areas in which improvements were noted.

The test scores of the Kentucky Core Content Tests were also reviewed to assess health education. These tests are administered at the end of every school year by the school per state regulations. We looked at the results of the practical living section of this test because this section assesses students' knowledge of health behaviors. Test results were ranked using three categories: novice for the lowest scores, apprentice for the middle, and proficient/distinguished for the highest. A paired-samples t test was used to test for differences between baseline practical living scores (pre-GSNC clinic) and current practical living scores at the schools in which a GSNC health education is provided (four elementary schools) (Table 1). The t test was significant with $P<.05$ for the change in number of students scoring at the apprentice level. The t test was also significant at $P<.10$ for the change in students scoring at the novice level. The shift in test scores is a positive one with students who scored at the novice level moving up to apprentice and those at

Table 1
Practical living scores paired-samples *t* test

| | Paired differences | | | 95% CI of the difference | | | | Significance (2-tailed) |
	Mean	SD	Standard error of the mean	Lower	Upper	*t*	df	
Baseline novice to recent novice	14	9.309	4.655	−.813	28.813	3.008	3	.057
Baseline apprentice to recent apprentice	9.5	4.203	2.102	2.812	16.188	4.520	3	.020
Baseline proficient to recent proficient	−15	21.618	10.809	−49.399	19.399	−1.388	3	.259

apprentice moving up to the proficient/distinguished level. Students who were already at the proficient/distinguished level stayed at that level.

Although these two evaluative examples give an indication that the presence of the GSNC in the at-risk schools may be making a difference, it is recognized that this is a natural environment and there may be other variables influencing the outputs as described in these examples.

Summative evaluation

The three concentric circles of the model surround and embrace the summative evaluation variables of effectiveness, impact, and sustainability. The following sections highlight our findings in each of these areas.

Geo-mapping analysis: effectiveness

To date, the analysis of effectiveness has been limited to an evaluation of meeting the primary health care needs of the children in the four elementary schools served by the Center. The technique of geo-mapping was used to provide a picture of how effective the project has been in reaching the children otherwise unserved by the health care system. Although geo-mapping is often used for planning it can also be used to assess the impact of a project.

The purpose of the geo-mapping analysis was to determine whether the GSNC school-based clinics serve children who are medically underserved, thereby validating the need for school-based clinics. Furthermore, this analysis investigated possible reasons that students who do not live in designated medically underserved areas (MUAs) still use the school clinics.

Geographic information system (GIS) technology is used to organize spatial data into a form that can be easily analyzed [18]. Using GIS technology, data from an Excel worksheet can be imported into the GIS software and coded to appear on the selected map. Geo-mapping is the term often used to describe the making of these data-specific maps.

The maps for this analysis were created using ArcView 9.1 GIS software developed by Environmental Systems Research Institutes, Inc. The geographic file of Fayette County census tracts was downloaded from the US Census Bureau's Cartographic Boundary Files Web site in the form of a Topologically Integrated Geographic Encoding and Referencing 2000 shapefile [19]. Individual census tracts were then coded by medically underserved area or distressed census tracts. Fayette County, Kentucky, has 17 census tracts that are designated as MUAs [20]. There are nine distressed census tracts in Fayette County, characterized by poverty rates significantly higher than national averages [21].

School and student addresses were plotted on a map of the county with medically underserved and distressed census tracts highlighted. The sample consisted of all students who had parental consent to be seen in the GSNC clinic who actually used the clinic at least once between August 2008 and

March 2009. Addresses were de-identified to protect the identity of the
students. Fig. 3 displays the map that was created showing where GSNC
clinic users live in relation to the medically underserved and distressed census tracts in Fayette County, Kentucky.

For the four elementary schools included in the analysis, an average of
24% of the population lived in an MUA, ranging from 0% to 71% for individual schools. One percent of the population lived in distressed census
tracts, ranging from 0% to 3% for individual schools. Additionally, an
average of 4% of the population lived in a census tract that was both an
MUA and a distressed area, ranging from 1% to 13%. Table 2 displays
details of where students live in relation to the medically underserved and
distressed census tracts in Fayette County, Kentucky. Although two of
the schools did not appear in an MUA, these schools' populations are composed of a majority of children on the free lunch program (meaning

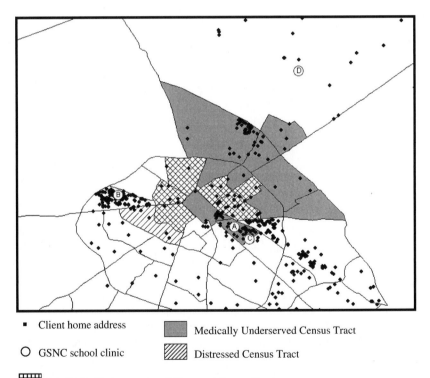

- Client home address   ▨ Medically Underserved Census Tract

O GSNC school clinic   ▨ Distressed Census Tract

▨ Medically Underserved and Distressed Census Tract

☐ Neither Medically Underserved and Distressed Census Tract

Fig. 3. Map of Good Samaritan Nursing Center school clinics clients in relation to medically
underserved and distressed census tracts. ■, client home address; ○, GSNC school clinic;
▨, medically underserved census tract; ▨, distressed census tract; ▨, medically underserved
and distressed census tract; ☐, neither medically underserved nor distressed census tract.

Table 2
Good Samaritan Nursing Center school clinic clients in medically underserved areas and distressed census tracts

Area	School A	School B	School C	School D	All schools
MUA only	41%	0%	9%	71%	24%
	n = 85	n = 1	n = 21	n = 113	n = 220
Distressed only	3%	1%	0%	0%	1%
	n = 6	n = 3	n = 0	n = 0	n = 9
MUA and distressed	13%	2%	1%	3%	4%
	n = 26%	n = 6	n = 2	n = 4	n = 38
Neither MUA or distressed	43%	97%	90%	27%	71%
	n = 89	n = 318	n = 207	n = 43	n = 657
Total	n = 206	n = 328	n = 230	n = 160	N = 924

individually they are underserved) (School B: 85%, School D: 68%) [21]. The other two schools also have a large proportion of students on the free lunch program (School A: 79%, School C: 51%) [22].

Based on the geo-mapping analysis, it was found that there are children in the GSNC school-based primary care clinics that come from areas of the county where there are no other services available to them. Furthermore, there are children who live in parts of the county that have health services. It is assumed that these services are not available to the children seen in the school because the children themselves live in poverty and are considered medically indigent. The GSNC school clinics serve not only as a safety net to children who have no other regular source of health care but also as an entryway into the health care system for students through referrals to other health care agencies. There are several reasons that some children do not have additional means of health care: (1) the health department is unable to fill all the needs of the medically indigent because of lack of resources, and (2) the Kentucky Children's Health Insurance Program (KCHIP) to provide health care coverage to children is not working as it was originally intended.

Nurse employment: impact

The last factor looked at when evaluating the Center was the nurses who have worked at the center and their current employment. Because the Center is an internship/fellowship opportunity for RNs (BSN prepared) interested in public health nursing and for nurse practitioners, there is an interest in learning where the nurses are employed after leaving the Center. In a survey of past interns and fellows it was found that 20 of the 30 RN interns who have been part of the GSNC are currently working in public health. That is 67% of the GSNC nurses working in public health, compared with 15% of the total nurse population nationwide working in public health. Furthermore, 10 of the 20 nurse practitioner fellows (50%) currently work in public health or in community-oriented primary care working with

vulnerable populations. Nationwide statistics for the number of nurse practitioners in community-oriented primary care working with unserved populations were not available for comparison.

Sustainability: partnerships

Although the Center has been extremely fortunate in having the work of
the Center recognized by the Good Samaritan Foundation as a worthy
endeavor that assists the Foundation in meeting one of its principle goals,
the future of the Center is predicated on the ability to sustain itself finan-
cially while continuing to meet the established goals. In 2007, an agreement
was entered into with the local health department to continue the four elementary school clinics and health-promotion activities and the one middle
school clinic. In addition local partners assist with continued support by
contract with the homeless clinic and the substance abuse clinic for homeless
women. Additional funds will be sought to continue efforts at the three free
clinics by providing support staff to those clinics.

Recommendations

To date the evaluation has included analysis of select goals of the Center.
The meeting of the primary health care needs of the children in four elementary schools has begun. There are numerous questions to be answered (eg,
Are there health status changes apparent in the children who attend the primary care clinics? Are the clinics the children's only means of health care?
Do changes in health behaviors knowledge translate into actual health behavior changes?). In addition, sentinels will be identified to determine health
status changes in the adults served by the Center. The model of nursing
practice in the Center seems to be a cost-efficient approach to providing
health care to vulnerable populations. The model needs to be tested by
cost-benefit or cost-effectiveness analysis.

Continued surveys of past interns and fellows will assist in determining
the impact the project has had on the workforce in public health and
primary care. Assessing the effects of the community partnerships and the
resource network to meet the clients' needs will provide data on the cooperative and collaborative efforts of the project. Most important is the impact
of the project on access to care.

Summary

The Good Samaritan Nursing Center seeks to improve the health and
health care access of vulnerable populations in Kentucky through its 10 primary care clinics, health education curriculum, and internship/fellowship
program. A geo-mapping analysis showed that the Center provides care

for children living in medically underserved areas and distressed census tracts. A simple cost analysis found that the services provided by the Center are done so through extremely reasonable costs. Attendance rates at schools with GSNC clinics are improving. The health education taught in the elementary schools has helped to improve health behaviors and state test scores. Most of the nurses working as interns and fellows at the GSNC have continued to work in public health or in primary care with vulnerable populations after leaving the Center, thereby improving the shortage of nurses working in these areas. It is obvious that alone this project cannot solve the problems of access to care for the populations served. Through the continued strength of the partners supporting this Center, however, a difference can be made. One of those differences is the level of awareness that has been raised by the Center director regarding the need to meet the Healthy People 2010 goal of a nurse for every 750 school children. Such a change in the primary community served by the Center will provide children an environment conducive to learning and to growing up healthy.

Acknowledgments

The authors thank the Good Samaritan Foundation, The Ministry of the Kentucky Annual Conference of the United Methodist Church, Lexington-Fayette County Health Department, the Fayette County school system, and the many community health providers for their encouragement and support. We also thank Dr. Juliann G. Sebastian for her work with this project and the Center.

References

[1] U.S. Department of Health and Human Services. Healthy People 2010: understanding and improving health. 2nd edition. Washington, DC: U.S. Government Printing Office; 2000.

[2] DeNavas-Walt C, Proctor BD, Smith J. U.S. Census Bureau, Current Population Reports, P60–233, Income, poverty, and health insurance coverage in the United States: 2006. Washington, DC: U.S. Government Printing Office; 2007.

[3] Institute of Medicine. Care without coverage: too little, too late. Washington, DC: National Academy Press; 2002.

[4] Institute of Medicine. Insuring America's health: principles and recommendations. Washington, DC: National Academies Press; 2004.

[5] Barger SE. Academic nursing centers: a demographic profile. J Prof Nurs 1986;2(4):246–51.

[6] Higgs ZR. The academic nurse-managed center movement: a survey report. J Prof Nurs 1988;4(6):422–9.

[7] Barger SE, Bridges WC Jr. An assessment of academic nursing centers. Nurse Educ 1990;15: 31–6.

[8] Tagliareni ME, King ES. Documenting health promotion services in community-based nursing centers. Holist Nurs Pract 2006;20(1):20–6.

[9] Sebastian JG, Stanhope M, Abu-Salem S. Organizational and environmental barriers to academic nursing practice. Proceedings of the Southern Nursing Research Society. 2004.

[10] Ritter A. Managed care credentialing and reimbursement policies: barriers to healthcare access and consumer chose. Philadelphia: National Nursing Centers Consortium; 2005. Available at: http://www.nncc.us/MCOProjectReportFINAL-wcoverpagev2.pdf.

[11] Hansen-Turton T, Line L, O'Connell M, et al. The Nursing Center model of health care for the underserved. Philadelphia: National Nursing Centers Consortium; 2004. Available at: http://nncc.us/NNCC_Publications/CMSRevisedExecutiveSummary120604.pdf.

[12] Institute of Medicine. Fostering advances in health care. Washington, DC: National Academy Press; 2002, p. 6.

[13] University of Kentucky. Commonwealth Collaboratives. 2005. Available at: www.uky.edu. Accessed March 13, 2008.

[14] U.S. Department of Health and Human Services. The registered nurse population: findings from the March 2004 National Sample Survey of Registered Nurses. Available at: ftp://ftp.hrsa.gov/bhpr/workforce/0306rnss.pdf.

[15] Good Samaritan Nursing Center. 2006–2007 Annual Report, University of Kentucky, College of Nursing, Lexington, Kentucky.

[16] Veney JE, Kaluzny AD. Evaluation and decision making for health services. Washington, DC: Beardbooks; 2004.

[17] National Centers for Disease Control and Prevention. Youth Risk Behavior Survey. Atlanta (GA): CDC; 2005.

[18] Gesler WM, Hayes M, Arcury TA, et al. Use of mapping technology in health intervention research. Nurs Outlook 2004;52(3):142–6.

[19] US Census Bureau, geography division, Cartographic products management branch. 2000 Census 2000 TIGER/Line Shapefiles. Available at: http://arcdata.esri.com/data/tiger2000/tiger_county.cfm?sfips=21. Accessed February 2, 2004.

[20] Bureau of Primary Health Care of the U.S. Department of Health and Human Services Health Resources and Services Administration, (2002). Medically underserved areas of Fayette County, Kentucky. Available at: http://bphc.hrsa.gov/databases/newmua/Detail.CFM?Combined_ID=01314. Accessed December 22, 2003.

[21] Appalachian Regional Commission. County economic status and distressed areas in the Appalachian region, fiscal year 2007. Appalachian Regional Commission. September 2006. Available at: http://www.gold.ky.gov/NR/rdonlyres/A86FCF1F-6FDE-4B45-AE77-AA46451F50A6/0/ARCCountyEconomicStatusDistAreasFY2007Kentucky.pdf. Accessed December 5, 2007.

[22] Fayette County Public Schools Office of Data, Research, and Evaluation (2004). Elementary school report for the 2002–2003 school year. Available at: http://www.fcps.net/sa/eval/2002-03-ES-Progress.pdf. Accessed March 4, 2008.

ELSEVIER
SAUNDERS

Nurs Clin N Am 43 (2008) 357–365

NURSING
CLINICS
OF NORTH AMERICA

Determining Standards of Care for Substance Abuse and Alcohol Use in Long-Haul Truck Drivers

Debra Gay Anderson, PhD, APRN, BC*,
Peggy Riley, RN, MSN

*College of Nursing, University of Kentucky, 315 CON Building,
Lexington, KY 40536–0232, USA*

Long-haul truck drivers, by standards of working conditions and work environment, are a vulnerable population. Long-haul truck driving is defined as driving distances that would not allow going home each night. Long-haul truck drivers deliver goods and services throughout the United States in addition to Canada and Mexico [1]. Drivers deal with job hazards that can increase stress levels and deplete coping mechanisms, that may lead to alcohol or drug abuse [2,3].

Few studies have been conducted dealing specifically with health issues faced by the long-haul truck driver. This vulnerable population is at risk for a multitude of health problems ranging from workplace violence to health issues, such as coronary artery disease and substance abuse [4]. This article deals with factors increasing the long-haul truck driver's risk for abuse of alcohol or drugs. Exploring this important topic uncovers factors that place the long-haul truck driver at risk for increased stress, that may lead to addiction. Finally, this article makes recommendations for standards of care that promote rapid identification of truck drivers at risk for addiction and for interventions for quick recovery to prevent long-term health consequences.

Background and significance of problem

There are approximately 9 million truck drivers in the United States, with approximately 3.1 million of these being long-haul truck drivers [5]. As a

Funding for this research project was made possible by the National Institute of Occupational Safety and Health grant R01 OHO7931.

* Corresponding author.
E-mail address: danders@uky.edu (D. Gay Anderson).

doi:10.1016/j.cnur.2008.04.003 **nursing.theclinics.com**

result of their job's description and characteristics, long-haul truck drivers are vulnerable to increased stress that can lead to abuse of alcohol or chemical substances. Increased stress levels have been found to increase the likelihood of abusing alcohol or drugs [2,3,6]. Identification of these factors that lead to increased stress is an important first step in identifying long-haul truck drivers at risk for abuse.

There are two major categories of risk factors that can lead to increased stress in the long-haul truck driver: work conditions and work environment. Working conditions include such factors as loss of support system, decreased amount of rest and relaxation, and decreased physical activity. Working environment includes such factors as driving conditions and workplace violence.

Work conditions

Long-haul drivers spend significant amounts of time, often weeks at a time, away from home and family. These extended stays away from home limit the truck driver's access to valuable support systems. Having a strong social and family support system has been identified as a buffer against stress that could lead to alcohol or drug abuse [2].

Working long hours may also lead to increased stress [7]. Drivers spend an average of 40.9 hours per week driving. Although the Department of Labor sets guidelines for driving extended hours, drivers must frequently drive beyond legal limits to meet delivery or quota deadlines for job security [1]. To meet delivery deadlines, drivers may turn to drugs, such as amphetamines, to keep them awake [8].

Sleep deprivation can quickly become an issue for the long-haul truck driver. Long periods of driving decrease the amount of sleep a driver can get and decrease the amount of downtime or relaxation time a driver can have. Adequate rest and relaxation are important as stress reducers and serve as protective factors against alcohol or drug abuse [2,9]. Compounding sleep deprivation attributable to increased driving time is the fact that high levels of stress can lead to insomnia, further decreasing the ability of the truck driver to get adequate rest [6,9]. Drivers may turn to illicit drugs and alcohol to help them get much needed sleep [8].

Little or no physical activity can also lead to increased stress. Physical activity releases endorphins, which act as a buffering agent against hormones that cause stress [2,3]. Spending extended hours driving does not allow the truck driver to have time for any physical activity. The most physical activity the driver may get is unloading or reloading the truck at delivery or pick-up sites [2,6].

One of the important findings that emerged from the study on Workplace Violence in Long-Haul Truck Drivers that can have an impact on addiction to alcohol or drugs is that of homelessness. Study findings suggested that a large number of long-haul truck drivers have no permanent residence; their truck is their home. Long-haul truckers, who are also without a permanent residence, are often faced with day-to-day survival needs, an increased risk for violence, increased stress, and decreased coping skills similar to those who are homeless and thus they are at higher risk for the use and abuse of alcohol and/or drugs than those truckers who have permanent residences [10,11].

Work environment

The work environment of a long-haul truck driver can be stress inducing. Truckers must drive in adverse weather conditions, such as rain, snow, or ice. Truckers must also drive at night or in high-traffic areas [1,5]. Sometimes, to avoid high traffic areas, truckers drive on weekends and holidays [1]. Truckers are also at high risk for road rage and other road safety hazards that can lead to an increased stress level [1,5]. Truckers spend a significant amount of time driving in strange and unfamiliar towns and cities. This factor places the trucker at an increased risk for violence, which can also lead to increased stress. Workplace violence is a major public health problem. In the United States, an estimated 20 workers are murdered each week in the workplace and approximately 1.7 million workers are injured each year from workplace violence [5]. Workplace violence contributes to 18% of all violent crimes in the United States [12]. The nature of the truck driver's job places him or her at increased risk for violence [5,12]. Certain workplace characteristics place victims at higher risk for potential assault and murder. These include having contact with the public; exchange of money; delivery of passengers, goods, or services; having a transient work environment; working alone or in small numbers; working late at night or early morning; working in high-crime areas; guarding valuable property; and working in community-based settings [5]. Long-haul truck drivers are subject to most of these risk factors at some point in performing their job.

It is important for public health nurses to be rapidly able to identify those at risk for potential alcohol or drug abuse so as to prevent long-term health consequences to truck drivers and their families. The study, Workplace Violence in Long-Haul Truck Drivers, has not only revealed valuable information about the risk of violence to the long-haul truck driver but other health issues that can have an impact on the long-haul truck driver. Sleep patterns, increased stress, and poor nutrition can have a negative impact on the health of the long-haul truck driver. Each of these findings needs further investigation to determine appropriate recommendations for interventions to decrease health risks to long-haul truck drivers.

Study methodology

In response to the need for accurate identification of workers at risk for violence, the study, Risks for Workplace Violence in Long-Haul Truckers, was carried out by Drs. Anderson, Reed, and Browning at the University of Kentucky. This was a cross-sectional, nonintervention study design using qualitative and quantitative methods. The study period was from 2003 through 2006, and the study was funded by National Institute of Occupational Safety and Health (R01 OHO7931).

The study aimed (1) to identify the types of violence that women and men experience while working as a long-haul truck driver; (2) to identify risk factors that contribute to violence against truckers and between truckers; (3) to differentiate the risks for work-related stress among distinct sociodemographic groups of truckers as they relate to specific exposures experienced by long-haul truck drivers; (4) to determine the prevalence of domestic violence experienced by long-haul truck drivers while driving when their driving partner is their intimate partner; and (5) to identify work environment factors that place truck drivers' safety at risk. Project aims were consistent with Healthy People 2010 objectives addressing reduction in work-related homicides (objective 20.5) and work-related assaults (objective 20.6), and with the National Institute for Occupational Safety and Health National Occupational Research Agenda (NORA) objectives.

The target population for this study was male and female long-haul truck drivers. Power analysis was used to determine sample size. A total of 987 male and female truck drivers from across the United States participated in this study. Recruitment occurred at truck shows and truck stops across the United States using a convenience sample of truck drivers. Because this job position is transient by nature, it was essential to go to the workplace to obtain data. Inclusion criteria for the study were commercial drivers who spend most work hours as long-haul truck drivers, age of 21 years or older, and ability to speak English. Long-haul truck drivers were defined as those who spend one or more nights away from home. Drivers also had a current commercial driver's license (CDL).

Measures

Participants completed a questionnaire designed by the research team entitled the "Work-Related Safety and Violent Victimization Survey." Questions on the survey related to work safety. In addition, the following scales were used:

- Conflict tactics scale. This was used to measure reasoning, verbal aggression, and violence within relationships. A seven-point Likert scale was used to self-report.
- Worksite harassment assessment measured worksite harassment.
- Trucker strain monitor used a Likert scale to measure work-related fatigue and sleep problems.
- Perceived stress scale measured life stresses.
- CAGE assessment measured drug and alcohol problems (CAGE is an acronym formed by taking the first letter of key words from each of the four questions: cut out, annoy, guilty, and eye opener).

- Demographic characteristics were assessed, such as age, gender, years driving, and socioeconomic factors.

Procedures

Qualified members of the research team or designees collected data at truck shows. Each survey took approximately 20 to 30 minutes to complete. Data collectors were trained in survey techniques and certified research integrity. Subject recruitment took place at truck shows, including those in Boston, Dallas, Louisville, and Las Vegas. Truck stops used for recruitment were located in Portland, Chicago, Des Moines, and two sites in Kentucky. Use of the various truck shows and truck stops ensured that data were collected from across the United States and reduced repeat individual participation.

Preliminary findings on alcohol and drug use

Preliminary study findings related to drug and alcohol use indicate the following: 63.04% indicated they had beer, wine, or liquor within the past 12 months; 38.79% indicated they had used alcohol less than one time a month; 36.82% indicated they had used alcohol one to two times a month; 14.12% indicated they had tried to cut down or quit drug or alcohol use; 2.87% indicated they had taken drugs or used alcohol to make things more manageable; and 8.25% indicated they became angry when someone suggested that they overused drugs or alcohol (Table 1).

Table 1
Preliminary study findings on drug and alcohol use by long-haul truck drivers

Type of use	Percentage
Had beer, wine, or liquor in past 12 months	
Yes	63.04%
No	36.96%
How often had alcohol	
<1 month	38.79%
1–2 times a month	36.82%
Several times a month	11.13%
1–2 days a week	11.29%
Almost daily	1.96%
Tried without success to cut down or quit drugs or alcohol	
Yes	14.12%
No	85.88%
Take a drink to make things more manageable	
Yes	2.87%
No	97.13%
Ever became angry when someone suggested you used too much	
Yes	8.25%
No	91.75%
Ever feel guilty or remorseful after drinking episode	
Yes	7.44%
No	92.56%

What the truck drivers are saying

Important qualitative data were obtained through one-on-one interviews with long-haul truck drivers at the truck shows and truck stops and through follow-up telephone calls to these truckers after they completed the survey. These qualitative data helped to identify issues faced by the long-haul truck driver that could have negative health consequences in addition to issues that indicated further investigative research. These findings also assisted in identification of specific risk factors that could lead to addiction of alcohol or drugs. Categories that have emerged from these interviews are social or family support system, safety, homelessness, availability of drugs, and job security.

Social or family support system

Several truckers mentioned the difficulties of being away from home and family. This causes loss of a social and family support system that can have negative consequences. The truckers are saying: "Our jobs take us away from home and family, and we are sometimes placed in dangerous situations"; "It's hard going days and sometimes weeks without seeing my family"; and "It feels like no one cares what happens to us as truck drivers."

Safety

Fear of victimization also places the long-haul truck driver at risk for increased stress, thus leading to alcohol or drug abuse. The truckers are saying: "As soon as I pulled up to the delivery site and got out of my truck, I was hit in the head with a tire iron; I thought I was going to die right there on the spot"; "Driving is dangerous; not only do you have to worry about road conditions, you have to worry about road rage"; "I have been run off the road many times by irate drivers, not truck drivers but other drivers"; "It is scary going to some of these places; you never know what is going to happen when you pull up"; and "The truck stops are as bad as some of the places I deliver to; you never know what you're going to encounter."

Homelessness

Homelessness has been identified as a significant factor for heightened risk of substance abuse and alcoholism. Without further research, it is hard to determine the exact number of homeless truck drivers, but interviews have revealed their existence. The truckers are saying: "My home is my truck"; "I can't give you an address because my home is my truck; all my belongings are in it, and that is not much"; and "Me and my dog travel together; we only got each other."

Availability of drugs

The ready availability of drugs can influence drug abuse. Truck drivers revealed how available drugs are at the truck stops. The truckers are saying: "When you pull up to a truck stop, almost immediately you are approached by prostitutes and drug dealers"; "I pulled up to a truck stop and before I could get out of my truck, someone was in the seat beside me offering me a pick-me-up"; "You can get almost anything you want at the truck stops"; and "I sometimes take something to keep me awake, not very often but just now and again."

Job security

Job demands on the long-haul truck driver create the atmosphere for increased stress. Truckers must drive long hours to meet company deadlines to keep a job. The truckers are saying: "Do you want me to put down the actual number of hours I drive or what I am supposed to drive"; "If I don't drive longer than the law allows, you won't have a job very long"; and "I have a family to take care of; if I don't drive, I don't feed them."

Nursing implications

In 2006, approximately 20 million Americans used illegal drugs and 17 million participated in heavy drinking [13]. Substance abuse and alcoholism have severe ramifications for the health of individuals and families. Abusers may ignore other medical conditions, such as heart disease, cancer, or mental disorders, to satisfy their addiction. Medical testing, such as radiographic imaging and blood tests, have found total systemic effects of long-term drug abuse [14]. Drug addiction may also place the abuser at an increased risk for engaging in high-risk behavior, such as unprotected sex, which can lead to sexually transmitted disease or HIV. Intravenous drug users place themselves at risk for HIV or hepatitis [14].

Health consequences of alcohol abuse include damage to the liver, cardiovascular system, immune system, gastrointestinal system, and skeletal system [15]. Alcohol abuse may also cause the abuser to ignore other health and mental problems. Abusers often ignore nutritional needs in lieu of alcohol, thus increasing negative health effects [15,16].

Safety concerns with drug and alcohol abuse also pose concern. In 2005, approximately 42,636 traffic accidents involved impaired drivers, with 16,694 of these being fatal [17,18]. The combination of lack of sleep, increased stress, and chemical impairment can pose a significant risk to long-haul truck drivers and those they share the road with.

As public health nurses, it is vitally important to develop standards of care for addressing these issues in this vulnerable population. Rapid identification of those at risk for addiction and quick intervention can decrease or prevent long-term negative health consequences.

Recommendations

The Workplace Violence in Long-Haul Truck Drivers study has assisted in identifying those drivers at risk for substance abuse. Recommendations for development of standards of care for interventions to meet the needs of this vulnerable population include increasing awareness of risk, making resources available, improvement of working environment, and policy changes.

Increasing awareness of risk

A campaign should be initiated to increase awareness of the potential of alcohol and substance abuse. Literature, such as flyers and posters, should be placed at frequently visited sites, such as truck stops, addressing signs and symptoms of increased stress, coping with stress, and stress reduction. Getting truckers to understand the importance of early intervention for stress reduction may prevent progression to substance abuse.

Resources

Placing information at truck stops with hot-line numbers and resource lists with health care providers trained in working with those at risk for substance abuse and those with addictions can assist the long-haul truck driver through early intervention. Early intervention, at the first indication of substance abuse, may prevent long-term health consequences that result from substance abuse.

Improvement of working environment

Improvement of the working environment should focus on providing truck drivers with opportunities for physical activity, improved nutrition, relaxation, and access to health care. Truck stops could be instrumental in providing truck drivers areas for physical activity and relaxation. Improving the nutritional status of truck drivers can be accomplished by providing healthier food choices at truck stops. Access to preventive health care, such as health screenings, could also be provided at truck stops.

Policy change

Stricter policies that focus on decreasing driving time that are aimed at operators should be implemented. Operators often place undue pressure on the trucker to increase the number of hours he or she drives in order to meet deadlines and maintain job security. Specifically targeting this group may assist the long-haul truck driver in getting home more often and allow for more downtime, therefore decreasing stress. Policies should also focus on the safety environment at truck stops and rest areas, making it safer for drivers to sleep and rest.

References

[1] Department of Labor, Bureau of Labor Statistics. Truck transportation and warehousing, 2007. Available at: http://www.bls.gov/oco/cg/cgs021.htm.

[2] American Institute of Stress. General information, emotional support and social support, stress in the workplace, stress reduction. 2007. Available at: http://www.stress.org.

[3] Brady KT, Sonne S. The role of stress in alcohol use, alcohol treatment, and relapse. Alcohol Res Health 1999;23(4):263–71. Available at: http://pubs.niaa.nih.gov/publications/arh23-4/263-271.pdf.

[4] Solomon AJ, Douchette JT, Gerland E, et al. Healthcare and the long haul: long distance truckers—a medically underserved population. American Journal of Internal Medicine 2004;46(5):463–71.

[5] National Institute of Occupational Safety and Health. Industry trends, costs, management of long working hours. 2004. Available at: http://www.cdc.gov/niosh/topics/workschedules/abstracts/dawson.html.

[6] Jerlock M, Gaston-Johansson F, Kjellgreen KI, et al. Coping strategies, stress, physical activity, and sleep in patients with unexplained chest pain. BMC Nurs 2006;5:7.

[7] Weiclaw J, Agerbo E, Mortensen PB, et al. Work related violence and threats and the risk of depression and stress disorders. J Epidemiol Community Health 2006;60:771–5.

[8] Davey J, Richards N, Freeman J. Fatigue and beyond: patterns of and motivations for illicit drug use among long-haul truck drivers. Traffic Inj Prev 2007;8(3):253–9.

[9] Haack M, Mullington JM. Sustained sleep restriction reduces emotional and physical well-being. Pain 2005;119(1–3):56–64.

[10] Anderson D, Riley P. The homeless population. Public health nursing: leadership, policy, and practice. Clifton Park (NY): Ivanov and Blue, Delmar Cengage Learning; 2008.

[11] Clark C, Rich AR. The relationship between alcohol misuse and homelessness, comprehensive handbook of alcohol related pathology. St. Louis (MO): Academic Press, Elsevier. 2004. p. 221–39.

[12] Centers for Disease Control and Prevention. Truck driver occupational safety and health, 2003 conference report and selective literature review.

[13] Substance Abuse and Mental Health Administration (SAMSHA). Latest national survey on drug use and health. 2007. Available at: http://www.samsha.gov/NSDUHlatest.htm.

[14] National Institute of Drug Abuse. Stress and drug abuse. 2005. Available at: http://www.nida.nih.gov/stressanddrugabuse.html.

[15] Roman PM, Blum TC. The workplace and alcohol problem prevention. Alcohol Res Health 2002;26(1):49–57.

[16] National Institute of Alcohol Abuse and Alcoholism. Medical consequences of alcohol abuse. Alcohol Res Health 2000;24(1):27–31.

[17] National Highway Traffic Safety Administration. Identification and referral of impaired drivers through emergency department protocols, February 2002, DOT HS809 412. Available at: http://www.nhtsa.dot.gov/people/injury/research/Idemergency/.

[18] Centers for Disease Control and Prevention. Impaired driving. 2006. Available at: http://www.cdc.gov/ncipc/factsheets/driving.htm.

ELSEVIER
SAUNDERS

Nurs Clin N Am 43 (2008) 367–379

NURSING
CLINICS
OF NORTH AMERICA

Promoting Oral Health Among the Inner City Homeless: A Community-Academic Partnership

Mary Lashley, PhD, RN, APRN, BC

Community Health Nursing, Towson University, 8000 York Road, BU116, Towson, MD 21252, USA

Homeless populations bear a disproportionate burden of oral health problems. Poverty, substance abuse, and co-occurring disorders render this population particularly susceptible to poor oral health. Racial, ethnic, and socioeconomic factors contribute to the disparities in oral health. Oral health care resources for the homeless are scarce, underfunded, and generally inadequate to meet the oral health needs of this population. Poor oral health has a significant impact on quality of life and may result in unnecessary pain and suffering; loss of self esteem; decreased productivity through lost days at work and school; difficulty in chewing, speaking, or swallowing; and even death.

The purpose of this program was to improve oral health among the urban homeless in a faith-based inner city shelter through education, screening, and improved access to oral health care. Funding was obtained through private foundations and charitable contributions. Collaborative partnerships were established with university dental and nursing schools, and volunteer dental care providers. Nursing students provided oral health education and follow-up shelter visits to promote appointment adherence. Dental students conducted on-site oral health screenings and provided emergency and comprehensive dental care through the university dental school clinics. Dental hygiene students also provided preventive care, education, and cleanings at the clinic. Residents were prioritized and referred for

The author gratefully acknowledges the following sources of funding support for this program: Abell Foundation, Leonard and Helen R. Stulman Foundation, Maryland Home and Community Care Foundation, and Baltimore Community Foundation.

E-mail address: mlashley@towson.edu

0029-6465/08/$ - see front matter © 2008 Elsevier Inc. All rights reserved.
doi:10.1016/j.cnur.2008.04.011

treatment based on pain, suspicious mouth lesions, and progress in the recovery program.

Since inception of the program 2 years ago, 279 residents have received oral health education. Residents have consistently evidenced a two to four letter grade improvement in oral health knowledge. Since program inception, 203 residents have received on-site oral health screenings and 218 residents have received treatment services, including preventive, restorative, endodontic, and periodontic care.

This program represents an innovative service delivery model and a collaborative cross-disciplinary initiative that is based on successful community-academic partnerships. Such a program can be potentially replicated in other communities to reduce health disparities and increase access to care for underserved populations. By proactively addressing oral health needs through prevention and earlier diagnosis and treatment, morbidity, quality of life, and cost can be positively affected.

Although nearly all oral diseases can be prevented, diseases affecting the mouth and throat continue to cause pain and disability for millions of Americans. Oral and pharyngeal cancers are associated with nearly 8000 deaths annually. Oral cancer rates are twice as high in men compared with women [1]. Most oral cancers are moderately advanced at the time of diagnosis. Poor oral health has a significant impact on quality of life and may result in unnecessary pain and suffering; loss of self esteem; decreased productivity through lost days at work and school; difficulty in chewing, speaking, or swallowing; and even death [2–5].

The first ever Surgeon General's report on oral health illuminated the serious disparities in oral health care among socioeconomically disadvantaged populations and the devastating consequences that result from such neglect. In the report entitled "Oral Health in America," then Surgeon General David Satcher described the importance of collaborative community-based approaches to fill the gap in oral health care [6]. This report was followed in 2003 by a National Oral Health Call to Action to promote oral health, improve quality of life, and eliminate oral health disparities [7].

Homeless populations are disproportionately at risk for oral health problems. Poverty, substance abuse, and coexisting medical illnesses and psychiatric disorders render this population particularly susceptible to poor oral health. Racial, ethnic, and socioeconomic factors contribute to the disparities in oral health. Among adults aged 35 to 44 years, twice as many African Americans as whites have tooth decay. The poor are at least twice as likely as those who are not poor to have untreated dental caries. African Americans are more likely than whites to have teeth extracted. Low education level is strongly correlated with tooth loss. Furthermore, oral and pharyngeal cancers tend to be diagnosed at a later stage in African Americans than in whites. The mortality rate from oral cancer among African American males is nearly twice that of whites. Together, alcohol and tobacco account for 90% of all oral cancers [1,2,8,9].

Unfortunately, oral health care resources for the homeless are scarce, underfunded, and generally inadequate to meet the oral health needs of this population. Challenges to accessing services include competing health priorities, financial barriers, inadequate transportation, and difficulty in navigating complex government assistance programs and benefits. Cultural, language, and literacy barriers also have a negative impact on knowledge of oral health [10]. Although clinics may exist to provide dental care to the underserved and uninsured, in many cases, partial payment is required to be able to access services. These fees may be cost-prohibitive for homeless clients. In other instances, services may be limited to cleanings or extractions. In some cases, the client must be receiving social service benefits to be eligible to receive care. Transportation to a source of care can also be a major problem for those unable to afford public or private transportation. At some clinics, it is not uncommon to have to wait several months before obtaining a dental appointment.

The overall Healthy People 2010 goals for oral health are to prevent and control oral and craniofacial diseases, conditions, and injuries and to improve access to related services. Related Healthy People 2010 objectives are (1) to reduce the proportion of adults with dental decay; (2) to increase the proportion of oral and pharyngeal cancers detected at the earliest stage; and (3) to increase the proportion of local health departments and community-based health centers, including community, migrant, and homeless health centers, that have an oral health component [2].

Purpose

The purpose of this program was to improve oral health among the inner city homeless through education, screening, and improved access to dental care. The program was conducted at a faith-based inner city mission and funded through private foundations and charitable contributions. Homeless residents enrolled in the mission's residential addictions recovery program received education on oral hygiene, signs and symptoms of oral cancer, and basic nutrition. Residents were screened for oral health problems by dental students and volunteer dental care providers. Those with priority oral health needs were referred to the dental school clinic for treatment. Services included preventive and restorative care, including cleanings, fluoride treatments, fillings, extractions, root canals, and prosthetics.

Program partners

Critical to the successful implementation of this program was the development of a collaborative partnership between a faith-based inner city mission, university schools of nursing and dentistry, and local dental care providers. Each provider or organization was instrumental to the success of this program.

The university dental school offered a wide range of educational and related professional programs and services. The dental school provided comprehensive dental care to the community through its primary care and specialty clinics. Dental students provided care within these clinics but also reached out to the community through the school's community cancer screening program. Under the direction of dental school faculty, dental students came to the mission to conduct oral cancer screening examinations and to triage for dental needs. Dental and dental hygiene students also provided preventive and restorative care within the academic center's dental clinics.

The participating mission was a nonprofit faith-based organization dedicated to providing hope to the poor and homeless through programs designed to meet the client's physical, psychologic, spiritual, and social needs. In addition to serving as an overnight shelter for the homeless, the mission housed one of the largest men's long-term residential addictions recovery programs in Baltimore. By partnering with individuals, businesses, churches, foundations, and other organizations, the mission provided a continuum of services, including counseling, medical, and legal services; vocational training; and job placement. Two years after graduation, 79% of graduates reported continued sobriety and 68% were employed [11].

Most residents at the mission were currently enrolled in the mission's 1-year residential addictions recovery program. Most residents of the program did not have access to dental care, and many had serious untreated oral health needs. The average age of mission residents was 38 years. Sixty-six percent of residents were African American. Seventy-two percent of residents were single. Fifty-eight percent of residents reported having at least one child. The average age of first drug use was 15 years, and the average length of addiction was 20 years. Seventy-eight percent of residents had a history of incarceration. The average length of incarceration was 34 months. Twenty-five percent of residents reported a history of mental illness. The primary drugs of choice were cocaine and heroin. Seventy-one percent of residents reported being enrolled in a residential rehabilitation program in the past. Two thirds reported having lost a job in the past because of their addiction. One third reported using Narcotics Anonymous/Alcoholics Anonymous (NA/AA) recovery resources in the past [12].

Because this population was in the process of addiction recovery, it was not uncommon for clients to experience relapse or to engage in behaviors that warranted dismissal from the facility. The mission had a zero tolerance policy for drug and alcohol abuse. Residents were randomly drug tested throughout the program. Residents testing positive for drugs or alcohol were terminated from the program and were not eligible to return for 6 months. Because this population had a high rate of attrition, measures were taken to ensure that valuable resources were not expended for care that was unlikely to be completed. This particularly applied to the manufacturing of dentures and prosthetic devices that were costly and could not be used by others should the client be terminated from the facility.

Therefore, in addition to having dental care providers assess the severity of oral health needs, mission program staff members were consulted regarding a resident's stability, progress in the program, and potential for recovery success. These factors affected the likelihood that a resident would adopt the oral health habits taught by the program for the long term, successfully follow through with referrals for care, and complete treatment. These factors were considered in establishing priorities for recipients to receive oral health care services. Residents with priority oral health needs (ie, pain, suspicious mouth lesions) and residents who successfully completed the initial phases of the program and who continued to live at the mission were eligible to receive preventive or restorative dental health care. Graduates of the recovery program in need of dental care who were in good standing with the mission were also eligible to receive services.

As a whole, the program represented an innovative service delivery model based on successful community-academic partnerships. Such a program could potentially be replicated in other communities to reduce health disparities and increase access to care for underserved populations.

Goals and objectives

The following goals and objectives were developed for the oral health program.

Goal

Mission residents would receive education on general preventive dental care and oral hygiene.

Objective

Student nurses would implement two mission-wide educational programs a year on oral health and hygiene.

Objective

At least 100 residents would attend the mission-wide oral health education programs each year.

Objective

Mission residents attending the oral health education programs would demonstrate a statistically significant improvement in posttest oral health knowledge scores.

Goal

Mission residents would receive screening for oral cancer and triage for basic dental needs.

Objective
At least 50 residents would receive oral health screenings each year.

Objective
All residents with positive oral cancer screenings or other serious dental concerns would receive a referral for follow-up care.

Goal

Eligible mission clients who were in need of restorative, preventive, or emergency dental care would access treatment services (ie, fillings, extractions, root canals, prosthetics, oral surgery, periodontal therapy).

Objective
Between 50 and 100 eligible clients who required follow-up care based on oral health screenings or who requested oral health care services would successfully access a source of dental care each year.

Objective
Eligible clients in need of funding for preventive or restorative care would receive funding for evaluation or treatment services (as long as funds were available).

Implementation

It was important to identify clearly the role of the staff, students, and providers in promoting project success. Nurses are integral to the provision of primary health care to the homeless. Student nurses also play an important role in addressing the health care needs of the homeless [13,14]. As part of this program, student nurses developed and implemented a mission-wide oral health education program to educate residents on risk factors, signs and symptoms of oral cancer, and basic oral hygiene. This intervention addressed a need to provide accessible and culturally sensitive health information. Nursing students also regularly visited the mission to address the health care needs of the residents and to follow up with clients scheduled for dental appointments, providing reminders of upcoming appointments and assessing any barriers to accessing care. Nursing students and staff tracked resident appointment adherence and delivered weekly reminders through announcements, postings, and verbal reminders. When possible, students followed up with clients who had missed appointments to assess the outcome of the visit and satisfaction with services rendered.

The staff members were responsible for coordinating appointments with dental providers, assisting clients to apply for eligibility for reduced fees, and arranging for transportation. To promote treatment adherence, services needed to be flexible, accessible, and delivered in a professional and supportive context [15]. To reduce barriers to care, residents who eventually obtained employment were accommodated through late afternoon and evening clinic hours.

To foster greater accountability, mission staff developed a written contract signed by the resident and witnessed by a staff member. The contract stipulated the nature of the commitment that the resident made to the oral health program and the expectations for keeping appointments or notifying staff of appointment changes or cancellations.

Dental students provided on-site oral health screenings and basic triage to determine priority treatment needs. In addition to the on-site screenings held at the mission, residents often presented to mission staff with emergent dental problems (ie, pain, abscesses). They were then placed on an emergency list, and an appointment with the dental clinic was arranged. Once emergency problems were addressed, if routine care was still needed, the resident was taken off the emergency list and reprioritized on a nonemergent list. Finally, residents with nonemergent oral health needs who were in good standing in the program and who requested an appointment with the dentist were placed on a waiting list for care. These clients were prioritized based on their progress in the program (eg, length of time in program, responsibility, accountability, commitment to recovery).

The waiting lists were in a constant state of flux and subject to reprioritization. For example, clients from the on-site screenings who were originally categorized as having urgent needs may have experienced an improvement in symptoms or located another source of care on their own while waiting to be seen. Of course, if the patient was in severe pain, he could be sent to a source of medical care to address his immediate needs (eg, antibiotics, pain medication for abscesses) until he was seen by a dentist. In the meantime, other clients may have presented with urgent problems that placed them higher on the list.

Services included comprehensive examinations, prophylaxis and fluoride treatments, emergency care, radiographs, extractions, root canals, crowns, oral surgery, and prosthetics (dentures) and were provided by students of dentistry and dental hygiene and by volunteer dentists. Many residents required multiple appointments to address their complex oral health needs.

Results

The program is currently in its second year of operation. To date, 279 residents have received oral health education. Residents have consistently demonstrated a two to four letter grade improvement in oral health knowledge based on pretest and posttest results. Since the program's inception, 203 residents have been screened on-site for oral health problems.

A survey of demographic data and risk factors was distributed to residents receiving on-site oral health screenings. Survey findings revealed that most of the population was black/African American (58% black/African American, 38% white, and 4% other). All participants were English speaking. No significant language barriers were encountered. The mean age of the population was 41 years (range: 22–61 years). One hundred percent of the target population was male. While 84% of the population reported having no dental insurance, 57% reported having no medical insurance. In addition, although most clients (69%) had not seen a dentist for an examination (not an emergency) in the past 3 years, only 34% reported not seeing a physician for the past 3 years (for nonemergency care). Moreover, only 14% reported seeing a dentist within the past year, whereas 52% reported seeing a physician within the past year for an examination (not an emergency).

Only 0.5% of clients reported ever having mouth or oral cancer. Clients did report having suspicious symptoms that could be suggestive of oral cancer (ie, lump or nonhealing sore in mouth [9%]; white or red nonhealing areas [6%]; difficulty or pain with chewing or swallowing [42%]; unusual bleeding, pain, or numbness in the mouth [28%]). Only 30% reported ever having a dentist or doctor look into the mouth for oral cancer. Of those who reported having such an examination, only 3% of these examinations were conducted in the past 12 months.

Tobacco use was common in the population, with 79% of clients reporting current use of tobacco in some form. Common forms of tobacco use included cigarettes (77%), pipe (2%), and cigar (2%). Sixty-one percent of clients who reported current smoking indicated they smoked less than one pack per day, whereas 13% smoked one to two packs and 1% smoked more than two packs.

Since program inception, a total of 218 residents have received treatment services. Of the 93 residents receiving on-site oral health screenings during the first year of the program, 31 were identified as having priority oral health needs (ie, pain, suspicious mouth lesions, significant oral pathologic findings). Of these residents, 55% successfully accessed oral health care services (defined as making and keeping an initial dental clinic appointment). The major reason for not accessing care was termination from the program (may be attributable to relapse, rule infraction, voluntary termination, or graduation and relocation). Of the 110 residents receiving on-site oral health screenings during the second year of the program, 27 residents were identified as having urgent oral health needs. Of these residents, 18 (67%) have successfully accessed care. The remaining 7 clients are still awaiting appointments.

All clients who were screened at the dental clinic received some level of oral health care; therefore, 100% of these clients were considered to have successfully accessed oral health care services. Treatment plans were established for clients seen in the dental clinic; however, some clients elected not to receive care or were terminated from the program because of relapse, rule infraction, or dismissal from the recovery program. In these cases, they were inactivated from the dental clinic patient list. Despite this attrition, the rate of client inactivation for this program in the second year was only 30%, compared with an inactivation rate of 50% for clients in the general dental clinic practice. Finally, 87% of residents who completed comprehensive restorative care were employed, 65% outside the mission and 35% as mission staff or interns (n=23).

Beginning in the second year of operation, residents were asked to complete exit surveys to evaluate their satisfaction with the program and the dental care they had received. To date, 18 surveys have been completed. All respondents agreed or strongly agreed that they were satisfied with the quality of dental care received through the program and that the program had enabled them to take better care of their mouth and teeth. In addition, most respondents agreed or strongly agreed that the dental care they received helped them to feel more confident (94%) and satisfied with their appearance (100%) and could even help them in the job market (78%). Moreover, most respondents agreed or strongly agreed that their dental care made it easier for them to eat (78%) and that they tended to smile more since receiving dental care (89%). One resident commented: "I'm so glad because I am now able to smile again. When I first came here, I had no teeth. Now I can smile with my dentures." Another responded: "I can eat! I don't look as old! Everything they did for me was great!"

Nursing and dental students were also surveyed regarding the impact that participation in this program had on their professional and personal development. Nursing students were asked to respond through journal reflections and dental students through e-mail communications and a Likert survey. Dental students (n=24) reported being more inclined to care for homeless clients (92%) and more sensitive to the needs of the homeless and underserved (96%). Moreover, students reported being more likely to consider volunteering their professional services to promote oral health among the underserved (100%) and more likely to advocate for the oral health needs of the poor and homeless (83%). Finally, students reported they would consider working in settings that provide care to homeless or underserved populations (100%). Narrative feedback provided further insight into this shift in thinking. Here are some particularly telling reflections from the dental and nursing students:

> Over the past few months, I have seen these men on a weekly basis. I always enjoy working with them because they are so grateful. I enjoy watching their oral hygiene progress, and I have come to understand that the encouragement that I can give them means so much because they are working so hard. These men have given me glimpses into their past and what they have struggled with, but I know that it is their past and they have put their past behind them and have turned their lives around. They recognize that part of getting their life back means that they need to take care of themselves, and have good hygiene. These men have impacted me so much, have given me great hope in the changes that can be brought about through [the mission], and I find great joy in helping them (dental student, personal communication, November 11, 2007).

When I first found out that my clinical experience would include working with this population, I was frightened and nervous. However, from the moment I stepped into the Mission I lost all of those feelings. The men at the Mission were extremely warm and welcoming, and relieved my previous worries that I had. I learned so much working with all of these men, and was inspired by each of their stories. I became aware of the fact that addiction doesn't discriminate and can affect anyone. Working with these men really gave me a chance to open my eyes and see that these men were people. They live and breathe just like everyone else... I feel as though I am more understanding and compassionate after working with this population. I have a deeper understanding of the challenges which many people face and the strength and courage which is required to overcome... Listening to the men share their views and life experiences was deeply moving... Overall I had a phenomenal experience...and learned more about myself than I ever would have imagined. I learned how to be a better nurse and how to be compassionate. I believe every nursing student should have the opportunity to experience this wonderful place... If given the opportunity in the future, I would love to volunteer and work with these men again (nursing student, personal communication, November 14, 2007).

Overall this has been a wonderful and fulfilling clinical experience. I will never forget the mission or the men I have met throughout this journey... Before working at the mission, I have to admit that I had a negative perception toward homeless people. The very first day after working with the men at the mission my perception about homeless people has reversed completely (nursing student, personal communication, December 5, 2007).

The men at the mission were not what I had expected. They were endearing and polite. They wanted our company and they appreciated the care we gave them... Overall going down to the mission is a blessing. It was the most meaningful clinical experience I have had. I think it was rewarding to everyone involved. I will miss visiting the [mission] and the magic that lives inside those buildings (nursing student, personal communication, December 12, 2007).

It really amazed me how much faith can change a person's life. As an individual, I have never been very religious but I have always believed in a higher power. But seeing how much faith has changed these lives has only made me want to learn more. I'm so thankful for all of the insight the men gave me. My family faces problems with addiction that I never really understood. Talking with the men helped me understand more and want to find ways to help my family members... As a professional, I will always take into consideration the person as a whole addressing physical, mental, as well as their spiritual needs. I love the [Mission!] (nursing student, personal communication, December 7, 2007).

Discussion

The program outcomes demonstrated the positive benefits of the program for the target population, students of nursing and dentistry, and participating organizations. By participating in the program, the students learned how to provide culturally competent care to a diverse underserved population. They also discovered the institutional, societal, and personal barriers that prohibit access to care for socially and economically disenfranchised populations [16]. This experience engaged students in critical reflection on the political and social forces that produce health care disparities and challenged them to make a difference in their communities of concern.

Students in the dental program had an opportunity to care for residents with complex oral pathologic findings. For example, one student shared with a resident that she was able to have most of her competencies checked off by treating just one patient, a feat rarely achieved! As a whole, the partnering universities realized a benefit by promoting the civic engagement of students in the community, a goal central to their missions. The mission benefited by receiving needed health services for its residents.

Finally, the program illustrates the value that can be derived from organizational and community-based partnerships. Faith-based organizations can effectively partner with academic institutions to meet community needs and to address health care issues of underserved populations. This program improved access to care for a high-risk population; at the same time, it prepared students in the health professions for community-based practice with at-risk and vulnerable populations.

The program provided for expanded delivery of oral health care services to the homeless. Access to medical care, in general, was far better than access to dental care as evidenced by the proportion of residents surveyed who had seen a doctor (52%) versus a dentist (14%) in the past year. Most homeless residents at the mission had little or no access to affordable dental health care. Residents with dental abscesses, for example, resorted to emergency room care when dental pain became severe and unmanageable. Antibiotics and pain medication were quick fixes that only temporarily provided relief. Many clients were in need of multiple tooth extractions and found that even clinics with low-cost or sliding scale fee schedules were cost-prohibitive. It was not uncommon for clients to seek emergency care for severe dental pain. This practice resulted in overuse of emergency rooms, increased costs of uncompensated care, and emergency treatments (ie, antibiotics, pain medication) that only temporarily resolved the problem.

Summary

According to the 2000 US Surgeon General's report, reducing oral health disparities requires a diversity of approaches that target improved access to oral health care for underserved groups and the population as a whole. Research is needed to evaluate the cost-effectiveness of oral health practices and the outcomes of oral health treatment for underserved communities [6]. For example, research on the impact of oral health care on self-image, stress, depression, social interaction, or employment would help to create a strong body of knowledge to address the effectiveness of oral health interventions on the population's health and well-being. Although research has demonstrated associations between oral health and systemic illness (ie, diabetes, heart disease), access to oral health care remains woefully inadequate for many underserved and vulnerable populations.

No longer can the mouth be divorced from the rest of the body. An intact smile promotes self-esteem, builds confidence, and creates a positive first impression that is particularly important for persons who have difficulty in finding employment and may have less than a perfect resume. By proactively addressing oral health needs through prevention and earlier diagnosis and treatment, morbidity, quality of life, and cost can be positively affected. Innovative, cross-disciplinary, community delivery models that involve key stakeholders at all levels are needed to address the oral health needs of the homeless and underserved.

Acknowledgments

The author gratefully acknowledges Reverend Keith Daye and the staff and residents of the Helping Up Mission in addition to Dr. Nancy Ward, Dr. Ed Grace, Patti Zimmer, Pat McGuire, and Christina Eckhardt from the University of Maryland Dental School, without whose contributions this program would not have been possible.

References

[1] American Cancer Society. Cancer facts and figures 2007. Atlanta (GA): American Cancer Society; 2007. Available at: http://www.cancer.org/downloads/STT/CAFF2007pwsecured. pdf. Accessed March 13, 2007.

[2] United States Department of Health and Human Services. Healthy People 2010: objectives for improving health. Oral health. Washington, DC: United States Government Printing Office; 2000. Available at: www.healthypeople.gov/Document/pdf/Volume2/21Oral.pdf. Accessed November 24, 2007.

[3] Huff M, Kinion E, Kendra M, et al. Self esteem: a hidden concern in oral health. J Community Health Nurs 2006;23(4):245–55. Available at: http://web.ebscohost.com/ehost/detail? vid=3&;hid=102&sid=eb32209f-0a49-995ad7f11. Accessed March 13, 2007.

[4] Oral Cancer Foundation. Oral cancer facts; 2007. Available at: http://www. oralcancerfoundation.org/facts/index.htm. Accessed November 24, 2007.

[5] National Cancer Institute. Oral cancer screening. Bethesda (MD): National Cancer Institute; 2007. Available at: http://www.cancer.gov/cancertopics/pdq/screening/oral/HealthProfessional/ page2. Accessed November 24, 2007.

[6] United States Public Health Service. Oral health in America: a report of the Surgeon General. Washington, DC: United States Public Health Service; 2000. Available at: http://silk. nih.gov/public/hck1ocv.@www.surgeon.fullrpt.pdf. Accessed March 13, 2007.

[7] Carmona R. National oral health call to action. Washington, DC: United States Department of Health and Human Services; 2003. Available at: http://www.surgeongeneral.gov/news/ speeches/oralhealth042903.htm. Accessed March 13, 2007.

[8] Centers for Disease Control and Prevention. National oral health surveillance system frequently asked questions. Atlanta (GA): Center for Disease Control and Prevention; 2006. Available at: http://www.cdc.gov/nohss/guideCP.htm. Accessed March 13, 2007.

[9] Centers for Disease Control and Prevention. QuickStats: percentage of persons with untreated dental caries, by age group and poverty status: National Health and Examination Survey, 2001–2004. MMWR Morb Mortal Wkly Rep 2007;56(34):889. Available at: http://www.cdc.gov/mmwr/preview/mmwrhtml/mm5634a5.htm. Accessed November 24, 2007.

[10] American Dental Association. Access to oral health care. Chicago: American Dental Association. Available at: http://www.ada.org/prof/resources/topics/access.asp. Accessed March 13, 2007.

[11] Helping Up Mission. Statistics. Available at: www.helpingupmission.org/lives/statistics.asp. Accessed November 24, 2007.

[12] Helping Up Mission. Helping Up Mission mid-year statistics. Baltimore (MD): Helping Up Mission; 2006.

[13] Wilde M, Albanese E, Rennells R, et al. Development of a student nurses' clinic for homeless men. Public Health Nurs 2004;21(4):354–60.

[14] Gerberich S. Care of homeless men in the community. Public Health Nurs 2000;14(2):21–8.

[15] Darbyshire P, Muir-Cochrane E, Fereday J, et al. Engagement with health and social care services: perceptions of homeless young people with mental health problems. Health Soc Care Community 2006;14(6):553–62.

[16] Treadwell H, Northridge M. Oral health is the measure of a just society. J Health Care Poor Underserved 2007;18:12–20. Available at: http://muse.jhu.edu/journals/journal_of_health_care_for_the_poor_and_underserved/v01818.treadwell.pdf. Accessed March 13, 2007.

ELSEVIER
SAUNDERS

NURSING
CLINICS
OF NORTH AMERICA

Nurs Clin N Am 43 (2008) 381–395

Transformation for Health: A Framework for Conceptualizing Health Behaviors in Vulnerable Populations

M. Christina Esperat, PhD, RN, FAAN[a,b,*],
Du Feng, PhD[c], Yan Zhang, PhD[d],
Yondell Masten, RNC, PhD, WHNP, CNS[b],
Seth Allcorn, PhD[e], Lorri Velten, MBA[f],
Lynda Billings, MFA[b], Barbara Pence, PhD[a],
Mallory Boylan, PhD[c]

[a]*Texas Tech University–Health Sciences Center, Lubbock, TX, USA*
[b]*School of Nursing, Texas Tech University–Health Sciences Center, Lubbock, TX, USA*
[c]*College of Human Sciences, Texas Tech University, Lubbock, TX, USA*
[d]*Department of Family and Community Medicine, School of Medicine,*
Texas Tech University–Health Sciences Center, Lubbock, TX, USA
[e]*The University of New England, Biddeford, ME, USA*
[f]*School of Medicine, Texas Tech University–Health Sciences Center, Lubbock, TX, USA*

Significance

The environment of contemporary health care in our society is fraught with complexity. The ever-increasing diversity of the populace and the continuous environmental change it engenders characterize this complexity. This is an inexorable process in which the burden of management of health behaviors under specific conditions becomes the most significant challenge of the health care researcher, planner, and provider alike. Accurate prediction and effective intervention in the management of health behaviors have been effected through use of known paradigms and models in practice and research. With increasing complexity and change, however, the limitations of these known paradigms and models in their explanatory utility have been exposed. In fact, various critiques of the power of single theories to

* Corresponding author. Texas Tech University–Health Sciences Center, Room 2B164, 3601 4th street, STOP 6264, Lubbock, TX 79430–6264.
E-mail address: christina.esperat@ttuhsc.edu (M.C. Esperat).

0029-6465/08/$ - see front matter © 2008 Elsevier Inc. All rights reserved.
doi:10.1016/j.cnur.2008.04.004
nursing.theclinics.com

explain health behaviors among diverse populations have been proffered [1]. Current thinking suggests that there is a significant need for new paradigms and models to be developed to explain health behavior more satisfactorily, particularly among high-risk and vulnerable populations in our society. Because these vulnerable populations experience a higher burden of health disparities, it is imperative that science provide stronger and more powerful theories and methodologies to explain how to predict and intervene in health behavior management.

Theoretic underpinnings: descriptive models of health behavior

Three categories of health behavior theories or models have been commonly used to explain and predict health behavior change at different levels: intrapersonal theories, interpersonal theories, and community and group level models. The most frequently used intrapersonal theories are the Health Belief Model (HBM); Theory of Planned Behavior/Theory of Reasoned Action (TPB/TRA); and stage models, such as the Precaution Adoption Process Model (PAPM) and Transtheoretic Model (TTM). Commonalities in concepts have been identified as these theories have been tested and refined. The concept of readiness is a central component of the HBM and TTM. Perceived risk is important in the HBM and the PAPM. Barriers inhibiting behavioral change are explicit in the HBM and TTM but implicit in the PAPM [2]. Self-efficacy, which is a predominant concept in Social Learning Theory and has been the most extensively tested in health behavior research, is embodied in these stage and process models.

The most frequently used interpersonal theories are the Social Cognitive Theory, Social Networks and Social Support, Transactional Model of Stress, Coping and Health Behavior, and Theories of Social Influences and Interpersonal Communication. The core assumption of these models is that people's interactions with their environments are critical determinants of their health behavior and, in turn, health outcomes. Their environments provide the means, models, reinforcements, resources, and sources of influence from which people gain information, skills, self-confidence, self-management competencies, coping behavior, and support [3,4].

Community and ecologic models of health behavior change have been conceptualized to explain levels of primary and contextual variables in health behaviors among individuals and groups further. Community and group models of health behavior change are the Theory of Organization Change, which focuses on mobilizing organization for health enhancement [5,6]; Media Studies Framework, with an emphasis on Communication Theory and Health Behavior Changes; Diffusion of Innovation model, which analyzes and explains the adaptation of a new innovation; and models used to improve health through community organization and community building. These models use the process of social change to investigate health behavior of populations and systems. Our society's most challenging public health problems require increased attention to organizational and environmental changes, provided that these changes are intensive enough and sustained over time. The Sociocultural Environment Logic Framework created by the Centers for Disease Control and Prevention (CDC) Task Force on the Guide to Community and Preventive Services [1] illustrates how community level factors influence behaviors but do not provide a multilevel approach. Application experience from planning systems, such as social marketing and PRECEDE-PROCEED, suggested that multilevel frameworks are more effective to help identify the appropriate social science theories that should be used in intervention.

Gaps in explanatory power of current models

Theories of health behavior have been shown to have predictive and practical value; however, there are also some serious limitations in the explanatory power of the most widely used theoretic models. For example, the HBM, which is focused on risk perception, has been criticized as being too far removed from the cognitive processes involved in the regulation of complex behaviors to offer a meaningful context with which to predict the interaction of multiple variables [7]. The model basically ignores cognitions that have been shown to be powerful predictors of behavior and fails to address the importance of external social variables, which can have a strong impact on intention formation (eg, the influence of others' approval on behavior). Because the theory does not articulate the anticipated relation between proximal and distal antecedents of behavior, there is a significant lack of explanatory power to bridge action-facilitation and regulation processes [7]. HBM research fails to explain how or which beliefs or cognitions mediate the effects of socioeconomic status in relation to particular health behaviors. This is particularly problematic in the attempt to understand how populations that experience significant health disparities act and make decisions about health. In essence, using an expectancy value orientation to explain behavior among vulnerable and high-risk individuals may oversimplify health-related representational processes. In other words, different operationalizations may or may not be strictly comparable [7] when confounding or mediating variables are expected to be operative.

Along the same lines, theoretic models of the proximal determinants of behavior describe how attitudes and beliefs determine behavior. TPB/TRA describes behavioral intentions, attitudes, subjective norms, and perceived behavioral control to explain behavior change. In essence, TPB focuses on perceived control by individuals in initiating and maintaining change behaviors. It has been pointed out that in the broad social environment, there are multiple influences on peoples' behaviors; thus, if the focus is perceived control, ignoring whether actual control is possible under certain circumstance, the use of theory to explain resultant behavior is therefore limited [8]. People who experience extreme burdens in overcoming environmental factors to change unhealthy behaviors may have little control over these factors. This is particularly true among groups that are overrepresented in health disparities populations. These explanatory models must pay attention to the broader social and structural factors that give rise to perceived and actual control problems if their utility is to be increased [8].

Stage models show progression of change behaviors through discrete stages. The TTM has been used widely by planners and providers of health care because of its intuitive appeal and because interventions can be easily developed around the focused constructs of the model. Questions still remain about whether stages are really discrete, however, and how behavior-specific these stages are [9]. Similarly, Bandura [10] argues that the Stages of Change and other stage models "substitute a categorical approach for a process model of human adaptation." Discrete stages may not adequately represent the rich complexity of behavior change. When interventions are focused on individuals and groups who experience serious disparities in health as a result of socioeconomic disadvantage, caution must be used in the application of these models to explain their behaviors and in planning stage-specific interventions without taking into account mediating variables that may have more explanatory power.

In the past several years, there has been increased attention to the larger environment in which behavior occurs. Some scholars have criticized a sole focus on individual health behavior as inappropriate. Others have suggested a broader focus on ecologic models that reflect the multiple levels of determinants of health behavior, and thus the multiple levels of intervention required to achieve the desired outcomes. Macrolevel approaches complement intrapersonal and interpersonal methods of health education and health behavior. Blended models suggest integrated strategies for reaching various units of practice in community-wide programs. Some health issues cannot be influenced through individual-level efforts alone. They may be affected positively, however, through methods based on individual-behavior analysis frameworks combined with two-way communication with public health leaders and media efforts to promote wide awareness and prompt community action. The integration of group, organization, and community intervention frameworks with individual and interpersonal models of health behavior has potential for a real-world impact that exceeds the use of any one approach.

Transformation for health: the need for an alternative paradigm

The transformation for health (TFH) is an alternative paradigm offered as an effective and parsimonious means of integrating constructs from multiple theoretic models that can be truly practical. Likewise, it can be used as a model that could lead to knowledge generation and testing. It is practical because it is intuitive and can be easily be used as a foundation for a broad view of system or community change at various levels in addition to being used for focused interventions in initiating behavior change at the intrapersonal or interpersonal level. At the same time, it can allow for substantial analyses of internal and external processes at those levels through formal research investigation. The parsimony of this model lies in the simplicity of the structural relational foundation of its basic concepts, which is easily comprehended and articulated. Nevertheless, it belies a complexity that allows for the integration and manipulation of multiple constructs from existing theoretic models.

The TFH has a philosophic and pedagogic base that is proposed particularly as a means of addressing the problems of health behavior management among populations vulnerable to health disparities. The TFH conceptualizes a transcendent process wherein people overcome oppressive conditions—whether these conditions are created through human design or from situational circumstances—that leads in different ways to the subjugation of the human spirit. Thus, this process is conceived to be primarily one that has to be made by the individual or entity enabling the self-transformation. The basic framework is founded on the ideas of Freire [11], a Brazilian educational philosopher who posited that individuals, people, or groups must achieve transformational power; it cannot be given to them. No one can empower another; self-transformation can only come from action within oneself [12]. It is a concept that hypothesizes the primacy of the person, whether individual or collective, in overcoming any condition that leads to the diminution of control and suppresses internal strength. This is a powerful idea that can be used in health care practice to assist individuals, families, and communities to transcend conditions that promote health problems and concerns deleterious to well-being. Thus, it has particular significance in understanding and addressing health disparities among vulnerable populations.

Philosophic and epistemologic origins of Freirean pedagogy

Freire's educational philosophy operates on the premise that disenfranchised people who are marginalized in society are victims of a type of oppression [11] that leads to disparities in their health and the health care they receive. The oppression is not necessarily human; for example, situations characterized by poverty, lack of education, minority status, and unemployment can be oppressive. Likewise, geography by itself can be a variable leading to oppressive conditions; persons living in remote rural communities can experience significant disparities in access to health care services that lead to deepening and prolongation of ill health [13]. Achieving transformation starts with the emergence of an essential element from within the individual, or the collective. Freire [11] refers to this crucial element in self-transformation as "critical consciousness," the ability to discern one's own realities, whether determined internally or externally. The emergence of this ability allows the individual or entity to move toward action in a process Freire refers to as "praxis." These two processes are elemental to the transformation process. Without critical consciousness, there can be no action; action without critical consciousness does not promote the type of transformation that overcomes the oppressive condition or situation. Because Freire's perspective was in the educational realm, he contextualizes this as a process of "liberatory education." Freire's philosophy is universal; its application has been replicated worldwide in many different ways and for various purposes.

The transformational process

Our organizing principle describes four sequential phases leading to the goal behaviors. Within these phases, multiple processes are conceptualized and can be designed for optimal explanatory value. Thus, phase and process are essential components in the explanatory power of this paradigm. In the cognition phase, the individual or collective will develops a critical consciousness that leads to a deeper understanding of inherent realities—an important first step in which the individual or the collective is able to comprehend the nature of conditions and the ways that they affect life. It also enables the realization that only he or she (or they) can control what can be controlled in the dynamics of transformation. Without it, there is no understanding that certain behaviors can lead to positive and negative outcomes of the process. With it, there is enabling of the evaluation of the resources that are available to make the necessary changes that optimize the positive outcomes and limit the occurrence of negative outcomes. The dawning of critical consciousness can be facilitated; this is where the helping professional can have an impact. Critical consciousness is a function of the epistemologic relationship that is built between the professional and the individual (or collective). This relationship is dialogical, which requires that the individuals (or entities) interacting within this relationship reciprocate in the cognitive processes to apprehend their own and the other's realities.

Development of critical consciousness is the first and primary element in this framework. Individuals range in levels of development of this state—from preconsciousness, characterized by magical and naive thinking, to full critical consciousness. People who simply apprehend facts and attribute to them a superior power by which they are controlled and to which they must submit, use magic consciousness. Those who see causality as static and use fanciful explanations and oversimplification of problems, whose thinking is characterized by strong emotional style and fragility of argument, are said to be in a naive state of consciousness. The critical state of consciousness is characterized by depth in interpretation of problems, by testing of findings and openness to revision, by avoidance of distortion and preconceived notions when perceiving problems, by refusing to transfer responsibility, and by rejecting a passive position [14]. It is in gaining critical consciousness that praxis—reflective action—is possible. In the health care relationship, it is an essential process to create an environment in which people can progress from earlier transitive states to full critical consciousness for movement within the transformational process to occur. The term *preconsciousness* is given to these earlier transitive states.

The process of critical consciousness development requires a relationship of knowing, an epistemologic relationship that Freire [11] characterizes as dialogical. This means that participants treat each other as subjects rather than as objects in a relationship that is horizontal rather than vertical, engaged in real dialog and communication, which is humanizing and makes every attempt at comprehending the other's realities. In essence, this requires an intersubjective space in which the dialog and communication can take place. In the health care relationship, this requires the health care provider, who frequently holds the balance of the power structure, to create a more balanced relationship and to take the health care receiver at the point of his emergence. This may also further require that provider demystification has to occur to create a more balanced relationship. Demystification permits less defensiveness and authentic availability of the health care provider to the health care recipient.

This leads to the intention phase, wherein the individual's (or collective's) motivational system is activated by the critical consciousness awakened during the previous phase to assess capacities for the transformative process and to develop the will to change. It is also during this phase that the individual or entity makes the decision to change the behaviors and the elements of lifestyle that lead to difficulties in controlling the advance of, for example, chronic disease and the multiple complications that lead to the comorbidities. A necessary element of the decision-making process within the individual or the entity is a firm understanding of the freedom to make choices from a set of alternatives. This is based on the understanding that although there may be others involved in the current reality, only he or she (or the collective) can make these choices. The dialogical process in the establishment of the relationship between the professional and the individual or entity can create this environment, in which choice and alternatives become clear. In the decision phase, the individual or entity actualizes the decisions that were made to change and maintain the behaviors that promote effective and successful self-management of negative conditions. It implies acceptance of responsibility for the consequences and outcomes of the decisions that have been made about the situation at hand. During the outcome phase, self- and guided evaluations yield evidence of intermediate, and possibly end results, of the actions taken by the individual to improve management of the process. The pragmatic elements of Freire's philosophy have particular appeal in working with disadvantaged groups, because direct involvement of the individual in the process of discernment and understanding of the circumstances that have led to the individual's (or entity's) oppression is required.

This framework is not intended to be a substitute for other theories of health behaviors. Its strength is not in its explanatory power regarding how health behaviors are formed or changed. Rather, its utility is in organizing thought about the basic nature of the health care relationship within which health behaviors are transformed. The TFH framework can be used to synthesize multidimensional constructs from the most common health behavior theories into a unified concept to describe the process by which health behaviors can be facilitated in practical and pragmatic ways. This makes it possible to generate testable hypotheses to discover whether and how specific interventions can be designed to facilitate peoples' efforts to overcome those health problems. This framework can be used as a model for exploring the mediational processes that underlie the complex relationships in health behaviors and the role that moderators play in effecting these processes [13].

The framework can be used to investigate variables at various levels of human interaction. For example, the achievement of critical consciousness can be examined at the individual and family levels, identifying factors that can promote or hinder the process at either or both of those levels. At the same time, it can model the development of a group's or community's awareness of the realities that may influence the health of members of the unit.

Operationalization of the transformation for health concepts

Individuals, families, or communities progress through the TFH model in a cyclic manner from the Preconsciousness state to the Transformational phase. The individual, family, or community may cycle through one or more of the phases more than one time before permanent transformation of behavior or praxis is achieved. Additionally, some individuals may not achieve praxis and spend most of the time in an earlier phase or cycling through earlier phases.

The schematic representation of the process is presented in Fig. 1, the TFH framework. The phases of the TFH are depicted as spheres connected by arrows in an incomplete circle, beginning with Preconsciousness and progressing through the Consciousness, Intention, Decision, and Transformation phases. Directional arrows on the schematic indicate progression of the cycling from phase to phase and between phases. Because Preconsciousness exists only until Consciousness has been achieved, recycling back to Preconsciousness or from Preconsciousness to any of the remaining phases for the same behavior is not possible. Thus, there are no bidirectional arrows from the Consciousness, Intention, Decision, or Transformation phases back to Preconsciousness. The process involved in progressing from one phase to the next phase occurs on a continuum and is identified by the name of the continuum between phases.

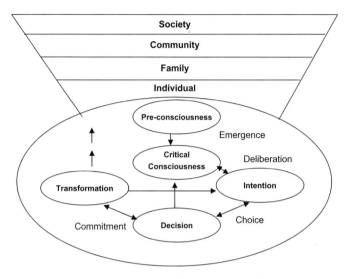

Fig. 1. TFH framework.

Definitions of each continuum identified in the schematic are as follows:

- Emergence Continuum is defined as the gradual progression from Pre-consciousness, indicated by transitive states of total or partial ignorance, to Consciousness, indicated by intellectual knowledge of, for example, less than "healthy" behavior. Along the continuum, the amount of knowledge increases along a steep curve until the Decision phase is reached.
- Definitions of each continuum identified Deliberation Continuum is defined as the gradual progressive transition from Critical Consciousness, indicated by acknowledging, "I would like to change a specific behavior," to Intention, indicated by stating, "I intend to change a specific behavior." The amount of knowledge continues to increase along a steep curve and peaks as Intention is reached.
- Choice Continuum is defined as the progression from Intention, indicated by beginning development of a plan for change, to Decision, indicated by completion of a full plan for changing the specified behavior. The duration of the planning process is determined by the sophistication of the plan and the availability or unavailability of resources for implementing the plan. The amount of knowledge peaks and begins decreasing along a steep declining curve until the planning for change has been completed and Decision is made.
- Commitment Continuum is defined as the progression from Decision, indicated by beginning implementation of the full plan for change in the specific behavior to development of a habit of changed behavior, or praxis, to Transformation. The amount of knowledge declines to

a plateau when the planning for change is completed when the Transformation phase is reached.

Causes of regressing, or recycling, to an earlier state include the emergence of new barriers or increased emphasis of old barriers. Table 1 provides an example indicating some of the barriers to progression (or maintenance of the habit once formed) and of promoters of progression through the transformational process, categorized according to individual context, in a particular situation.

Case application for operationalization of the transformation for health at the individual level

The use of the TFH can be demonstrated by use of a case example at the individual level. The client in the case example is a 45-year-old, low-socioeconomic, male client who is employed in a minimum-wage warehouse laborer position and has been smoking since the age of 13 years. There are no employment restrictions to smoking "on the job." All male friends and family members smoke. Currently, the client smokes at least two packs of cigarettes each day. Because of employer requirements, the client is being seen at a local community health clinic for an annual assessment. No health

Table 1
Transformation for health: example of individual contextual factors impeding or promoting movement through the process

Individual context	
Barriers	Promoters
Situational context	
Physical (capability to access information for implementing decision)	
Addiction	Pharmaceutic aids
Physical inability to access additional resources	Help with planned recovery
Financial (annual income, resources)	
Limited finances for change	Free information
	Free programs
	Increase in personal funds
Educational (education level of achievement, ability to understand information)	
Low health literacy	Access to additional information
	Clarification of benefits of nonsmoking
Employment (work, occupation)	
No incentives	Financial, through continued employment
Psychologic context (mental and emotional factors)	
Compulsions (addiction)	Projection of success (fantasy)
Problem recognition	Guided imagery
Relational context (personal and interpersonal relationship factors)	
Lack of support (family, peers, coworkers, employer)	Positive role models
	Positive social support

care provider has discussed smoking cessation or the negative impact of smoking on health status.

In the Preconsciousness state of the TFH, the client is unaware of the negative health consequences of smoking. Additionally, the client has no health care prevention or health promotion plan, no exercise regimen other than working in a warehouse, and visits a health care provider only when an illness is severe enough to prevent working. At the annual assessment appointment, the nurse practitioner begins the process of exploring with the client his years of smoking experience—gaining from his point of view the realities in his life that first led him to smoking and then sustained that experience. The practitioner does not start out the relationship by pointing out the negative health consequences of smoking at least two packs of cigarettes a day for 32 years. The barriers and promoters are presented in Table 1. The practitioner assists the client to identify potential barriers that lead to continuation of the smoking habit and promoters for progression through the transformational process. During the physical assessment, the practitioner then continues by presenting to the client physical evidence of the negative impact of smoking for the client. At the follow-up visit, the nurse practitioner is able to show how the laboratory and radiographic results document the negative health consequences of smoking. Nevertheless, the client is not willing, or not able, to make a decision for smoking cessation at this point; the practitioner does not push him to make that decision.

During the Critical Consciousness phase of the TFH, the client is able to describe to the nurse practitioner the negative consequences of smoking. The client is still unable to make the decision to stop smoking; the practitioner does not impose any pressure on the client to make that decision. During a follow-up visit for employer-required flu immunization, the nurse practitioner revisits with the client the benefits to be gained by quitting the habit. The Intention phase of the TFH is evident in the second annual assessment visit to the community health clinic. The client and nurse practitioner once again revisit and discuss the barriers that possibly impede the client's progress in this process. The practitioner further reinforces the need to quit by helping him to identify other promoters that the client may still not be aware of. The client moves to the Decision phase, resolves to quit smoking, and works with the nurse practitioner to design an individualized smoking cessation plan. A follow-up visit is scheduled for 3 months later. At the follow-up visit, the client shares his success in stopping smoking for 2 months; however, he then attended a family event at which all his male friends and relatives were smoking, and he therefore "relapsed." Thus, the client has cycled back to the Critical Consciousness phase. Over the next 6 months, the client and nurse practitioner work to successfully move the client back to the Intention phase.

At the annual assessment visit 2 years later, the client has been smoke-free for 18 months and is free of the physical craving but not the emotional craving for a cigarette. The barriers remain evident, but the client is clearly demonstrating the process of progression through the Transformational Behavior phase. The client may or may not be able to move to the final Transformational Behavior phase, wherein a permanent change has occurred when the client has established continuous smoking cessation behavior and there are no situations capable of tempting the client to relapse into smoking again. As long as the client has not reached this final phase, there remains the potential for the client to relapse and cycle back to the earlier phases and for him to stay in those intermediate phases.

Case application for operationalization of the transformation for health at the community level

A community coalition for health improvement is formed by three leaders representing a community center, an academic nurse-managed primary care center, and an elementary school located in one of the most economically disadvantaged areas of the city, where the Hispanic population predominates. Some of the coalition members have heard that one of the problems experienced by community residents is the high incidence of childhood obesity in the neighborhood schools within the area. In the process of gaining Critical Awareness of their situation, the coalition undertakes a community needs assessment to understand the problem more thoroughly. As the members of the coalition move through the Emergence Continuum, they learn that, indeed, the incidence of obesity and overweight is significantly higher among the fifth graders in the neighborhood elementary school and that the parents of the children, in addition to other community residents, did perceive overweight and obesity to be a problem among the school children. In addition, they learned that certain barriers exist that predispose to the problem: lack of safe areas for children to play; limited finances to buy more nutritious meals, such as fruits and vegetables; and too much unsupervised television watching among the children. They also learn that they have one of the most potent promoters for change: the resolve and dedication of the members of the coalition to change their conditions. Thus, they move through the Deliberation Continuum into the Intention phase of the Transformation process by determining to work together to change the conditions in the community. The principal of the elementary school helps to raise funds for an outdoor learning center in his school, where children can play and build gardens. The administrator representing the academic nurse-managed primary care center pulls together a team to respond to a request for proposals for research projects focusing on human nutrition and obesity. The community center provides the place for coalition meetings and supports the initiatives in different ways. Thus, the coalition progresses to Decision through the Choice Continuum to tackle this particular community problem.

The outdoor learning center is slowly built, as funds are gathered. The research proposal was submitted, and although the submission was not successful the first time, the coalition persisted and continued to support the project team in a successful resubmission, resulting in 3 years of significant funding for an integrated project to implement nutrition, physical activity, and gardening curricula in the early grades before the children get to the fifth grade. The community center obtained funding to provide summer programs of physical activities and healthy lunches to the school children during the summer break. Together, the coalition participants learned as they moved through the Commitment Continuum that community Transformation can only come with the knowledge and understanding of the barriers and promoters to change that they face and with their own efforts at achieving transformational behaviors that lead to change.

Discussion

Both of these cases attempt to show the constructs applied at the specified levels of operationalization. The individual-level application illustrated movement between phases and cycling back to earlier phases. The dialogical relationship that was established between the helping professional and the client meant that the individual was a subject rather than an object in terms of the interactions that took place and that the professional made the effort to lessen the intersubjective distance that characterized their communications by providing assistance in identifying the barriers and promoters to the individual's circumstances and yet, at the same time, allowing him to make progress at his own pace and on his own terms, thus helping the professional to keep the client engaged in the process. The professional recognized that starting out the relationship by pressuring him to quit a negative behavior did not recognize that client's need to develop a critical awareness of his own realities relative to the smoking experience and would have been counterproductive to the process. Instead of pressure, the professional used facilitation of the environment to move the client through the process.

In the community situation, the critical consciousness was arrived at collectively through a community needs assessment process using structured methods of gathering information regarding the community's realities relative to the pressing needs and problems experienced by the collective. The group guided themselves through the Transformational process, through their sustained interactions and through the relation of communications and commitment to common goals.

Although they differ in terms of the circumstances of occurrence and the outcomes of the process, the progression between phases at these two levels follow similar trajectories. Whereas the individual-level application illustrated the facilitation by a helping professional who worked with the individual to raise his critical consciousness to the point of being able to move to the next phase in the process, the community worked together as a collective toward raising its own level of critical consciousness and moved as an entity toward transformational behavior.

Summary

As the case illustrations show, raising critical consciousness of people's or communities' realities within their environments is the starting point for action. Individuals or groups have to be able to assess successfully the influence of psychosocial or cultural factors that influence their individual realities and their impacts on specific situations or on their lives in general. Critical consciousness is a powerful antecedent to intention and decision. Interventions can be designed to foster or enhance this phenomenon, particularly among people who are marginalized by circumstances beyond their control. Systematic testing of the effectiveness of these interventions can be conducted, focusing particularly on the mediating and moderating variables that exert their subtle and complex impacts on the relations among the primary variables [13]. The knowledge gained through these systematic investigations could yield potent ammunition for advocacy for program development and public policy changes.

Shedding light on the factors and circumstances that operate to bring about marginalization of groups can facilitate appropriate responses to the issue of health disparities among vulnerable groups in society. This is showing to be a seemingly intractable problem; however, it may well be that the approaches currently used to respond to the issues are not appropriate because we overlook the "realities" that really matter: those emanating from the people being visited by these circumstances themselves. Until we realize that pouring information and resources on problems can be counterproductive unless peoples' realities are known and taken account of, we are likely to continue to spin our wheels on the same problems. Under normal conditions, human behavior can only be controlled by the individual. Facilitating an environment in which an individual can comprehend his or her internal and external realities is the first step toward transformative behavior.

References

[1] National Cancer Institute. Theory at a glance: a guide for health promotion practice. National Institutes of Health; 2005. Available at: http://www.cancer.gov/PDF/481f5d53-63df-41bc-bfaf-5aa48ee1da4d/TAAG3.pdf.

[2] Rimer B. Perspectives on intrapersonal theories of health behavior. In: Glanz K, Rimer BK, Lewis FM, editors. Health behavior and health education. 3rd edition. San Francisco (CA): Jossey-Bass; 2002. p. 144–60.

[3] Glanz K. Perspectives on using theory. In: Glanz K, Rimer BK, Lewis FM, editors. Health behavior and health education. 3rd edition. San Francisco (CA): Jossey-Bass; 2002. p. 545–58.

[4] Lewis F. Perspectives on models of interpersonal health behaviors. In: Glanz K, Rimer BK, Lewis FM, editors. Health behavior and health education. 3rd edition. San Francisco (CA): Jossey-Bass; 2002. p. 265–74.

[5] Glanz K. Perspectives on group, organization and community interventions. In: Glanz K, Rimer BK, Lewis FM, editors. Health behavior and health education. 3rd edition. San Francisco (CA): Jossey-Bass; 2002. p. 289–404.

[6] Anderson LM, Scrimshaw SC, Fullilove MT, et al. The community guide's model for linking the social environment to health. Am J Prev Med 2003;24(Suppl 3):12–20.

[7] Sheehan P, Abraham C. The health belief model. In: Conner M, Norman P, editors. Predicting health behaviors. Philadelphia: Open University Press; 1998. p. 23–67.

[8] Conner M, Sparks P. The theory of planned behavior and health behaviors. In: Conner M, Norman P, editors. Predicting health behaviors. Philadelphia: Open University Press; 1998. p. 121–62.

[9] Glanz K, Rimer BK, Lewis FM. Health behavior and health education: theory, research, and practice. 3rd edition. San Francisco (CA): Jossey-Bass; 2002.

[10] Bandura A. Health promotion from the perspective of social cognitive theory. In: Norman P, Abraham C, Conner M, editors. Understanding and changing health behaviour. Reading (UK): Harwood; 2000. p. 299–339.

[11] Freire P. Pedagogy of the oppressed. New York: The Continuum International Publishing Group; 1970.

[12] Esperat MC, Gilmore P, Dorsey-Turner G. Transformative power: healing the wounds of cultural oppression. In: Kritek P, editor. Reflections on healing: a central nursing construct. New York: NLN Press; 1997. p. 224–33.

[13] Esperat MC, Feng D, Owen D, et al. Transformation for health: a framework for health disparities research. Nurs Outlook 2005;53(3):113–20.

[14] Freire P. Education for critical consciousness. New York: The Continuum International Publishing Group; 1973.

ELSEVIER
SAUNDERS

NURSING
CLINICS
OF NORTH AMERICA

Nurs Clin N Am 43 (2008) 397–417

Translating Research on Healthy Lifestyles for Children: Meeting the Needs of Diverse Populations

Christine Kennedy, RN, CPNP, PhD, FAAN*,
Victoria Floriani, RN, CPNP, APRN-BC

*Department of Family Health Care Nursing, University of California,
2 Koret Way, Box 0606, San Francisco, CA 94143–0606, USA*

Poor health consequences in children are often related to lifestyle factors rather than to disease processes. An expansive literature has emerged that describes the rapidly deteriorating and interrelated nature of health risk behaviors in American children and youth. The data indicate that half of school-aged children are at moderate risk for engaging in two or more risk behaviors [1]. Categoric risk-taking behaviors include substance use, early sexual activity, delinquency, violent behaviors, school failure, and mental health problems associated with depression and stress. Injuries, as an outcome of risky behavior, are among the leading causes of death in children aged 1 to 18 years [2]. In addition, poor nutritional habits, increased sedentary behavior, and lack of physical activity (PA) among children have been linked to increasing obesity rates, with 17% of the nation's children aged 2 to 19 years being overweight in 2004 [3].

Studies of children's health beliefs, perceptions, and practices have documented that children's health-compromising behaviors generally cluster, increase as children get older, and are relatively well defined and stable by 9 to 11 years of age. The 2005 national Youth Risk Behavior Survey (YRBS) [4] found that adolescents in the month preceding the survey were engaging in

---

This work was partially supported by a grant from the National Institutes of Health/National Institute of Nursing Research (1 RO1 NR04680-01A2) "Prevention Interventions in Hispanic and Anglo Children" and from the Health Resources and Services Administration (07-40314 NEPR) "Improving Health Equity for Children and Families."

* Corresponding author.

E-mail address: christine.kennedy@nursing.ucsf.edu (C. Kennedy).

doi:10.1016/j.cnur.2008.04.001
nursing.theclinics.com

alcohol consumption (43%), cigarette smoking (23%), physical fighting (36%), and sexual intercourse (47%), among other health risk behaviors. Homicide climbs to the rank of the second greatest killer of teens aged 15 to 18 years, with firearms as the leading method [3]. The highest rates of obesity and overweight among children in 2004 were in the 6- to 11-year-old age group at almost 19%, followed by adolescents (12–19 years of age) at 17% [2]. These data highlight the early school-aged years as a critical period for interventions directed toward reinforcing healthy lifestyle behaviors.

One cannot discuss trends in the health behaviors of children without taking into account socioeconomic variables. Census data from recent years show that in the United States, more than 40% of children younger than the age of 18 years come from diverse racial and ethnic backgrounds. Approximately 20% of children in the United States are Hispanic, 17% are African American, 4% are Asian, 1% are American Indian or Alaskan native, and less than 1% are native Hawaiian or Pacific Islander [5]. These statistics are significant, given that in many cases, health behavior patterns tend to differ among children from different racial and ethnic backgrounds. In 2004, black and Mexican-American children aged 2 to 19 years had higher rates of overweight than whites (19% and 20% versus 16%, respectively). Black and Hispanic adolescents in the 2005 YRBS also demonstrated higher prevalence over their white counterparts in certain health risk behaviors, including physical fighting (43% and 41% versus 33% respectively), sexual intercourse (67% and 51% versus 43%), and time spent watching television (64% and 46% versus 29%) [4].

In 2005, more than 28% of US children were living in a single-parent household, with 50% of all black children and 25% of all Hispanic children living with a single mother [6]. Single-mother households in the United States carried the highest family poverty rates in 2006, with 28% living lower than the poverty line [7]. Almost 12% of all US children in 2006 had no health insurance coverage, and the numbers were even more dismal for minority children, with 22% of Hispanic children and 14% of black children uninsured [7].

These grim statistics support concern for the continuing effects of disparities in health in the pediatric population. Given the negative trajectory and lack of improvement in meeting the Healthy People 2010 goals, translational efforts to accelerate the results of scientific findings into primary or community health are self-evident. Whether the recent National Institutes of Health (NIH) commitment [8] realizes its potential to shorten the time gap of this adaptation process and facilitate meeting the two Healthy People 2010 major goals for the United States to (1) increase the quality and years of healthy life and (2) eliminate health disparities [9] is critical for nursing to monitor.

The following discussion presents two different approaches to addressing two significant health lifestyle behaviors of children from vulnerable populations: television viewing and PA. Specifically the authors explore nursing interventions in the after-school environment and the primary care setting, two relatively understudied contexts for these areas of health yet highly accessible to reach diverse populations. In the first intervention, the authors review the design, implementation, and evaluation of a successful community-based after-school program aimed toward the reduction of television-influenced risk-taking behavior among children. In the second, the authors look at the design and implementation plan for a currently funded translational project underway in an inner city primary care setting designed to encourage and motivate increased PA among children and their families.

Intervention 1: after-school programs

Television as an influence on children's developing health behaviors

Health science researchers have well established that children's television viewing affects their health behaviors. Advertisements and portrayals of alcohol and tobacco use on television and in the movies have significantly contributed to youth drinking and smoking [10]. Media portrayals of unrealistically proportioned models have led to an increase in children's body image dissatisfaction, often leading to lowered self-esteem and disordered patterns of eating [11]. Media depictions of sexual activities without real-life consequences (eg, pregnancy and sexually transmitted disease [STD] infection) have been associated with an increase in youth perception of sexual activity in the real world [12]. Indeed, risk taking is portrayed in the media as free of consequences, with harmful outcomes depicted in only 3% of risky scenes [13].

There is a significant amount of evidence linking sedentary behavior to childhood obesity and overweight [14–19]. Combined with the increased sedentary behavior associated with viewing television, advertisements for high-calorie, high-sugar, and high-fat foods have contributed to 17% of children and adolescents aged 6 to 19 years currently being overweight [2], placing children at a greater risk for developing chronic diseases, such as heart disease and type 2 diabetes. Interventions aimed at reducing time spent watching television or other forms of screen time have been shown to lower unnecessary calorie consumption, decrease adiposity or body mass index (BMI) levels, or, in some cases, increase PA levels [18,20–27]. A 2-year long study by Motl and colleagues [28] found that a decrease in the amount of time spent by early adolescents (n = 4594) watching television was significantly associated with an increase in the frequency of leisure-time PA. Thus, interventions aimed at decreasing sedentary behavior are highly supported as part of a multidimensional program to reduce and maintain overweight in children [29,30].

Although the negative health consequences of children's media consumption and its associated developmental trajectories have been well researched, the socialization of children's health behaviors remains underexplored [31,32]. Although there are several historical descriptive studies regarding children's use of television, few studies have sought to approach children directly regarding their motivations for watching television. Researchers who have directly assessed children's motivations for watching television have found that children watch television as a coping strategy, albeit an ineffective one [33], and as a means for spending time with their parents [34]. Children also report perceiving television as a friend, with several researchers demonstrating that television establishes normative behavior much in the same way as a peer [34,35].

Previous intervention programs

Family- and school-based interventions aimed at changing the amount of time that children view television have reported some success. Jason and his colleagues [36–40] reported nine case studies that modified children's television viewing practices in households with young children (aged 3–13 years), all of which were effective. The approaches of these investigators shared the same strategy of the children receiving reinforcement for alternative activities. They noted that the use of mere "rules" in the households had been historically ineffective, particularly in households in which viewing hours were particularly excessive (>4 hours a day). Singer and colleagues [41] have also demonstrated that interventions aimed at changing children's viewing behaviors by working only with the subjects' parents were ineffective.

Two school-based programs have reported similarly positive results. Dorr and colleagues [42–44] indicate that children in kindergarten and third grade have been able to demonstrate appreciable change in their understanding of the effect of television content when they are instructed and have an opportunity to practice the new skills. More recently, Robinson [18] demonstrated that a school-based program was effective in reducing third- and fourth-grade children's television viewing time, BMI, video games use, and frequency of eating meals in front of the television. Robinson's intervention program was composed of 18 lessons integrated into the school curriculum, occurring over a period of 7 months. In addition to receiving the lesson, the intervention group budgeted their watching or playing time, practiced more selective use of play, and received limited access to television.

Theoretic model

Based on the findings of the authors' own pilot work [34], they created a program aimed at limiting media influence on the development of adverse risk-taking and dietary behaviors in young school-aged children. In contrast to the interventions reported here, the authors' program was less reliant on parental involvement or the external application of parental rules. Further, it was less time- and resource-intensive and was easily replicated by trained staff in after-school programs and community-based sites.

To understand how children understand and respond to television and how television influences their risk-taking and dietary behaviors, children's viewing experiences must be considered from a developmental perspective and within a larger social context. Guided by motivational and self-change theories [45,46], the Kids TV Study intervention uses a behavioral approach to change children's television habits and self-care behaviors.

The intervention program postulates television as a potentially modifiable social influence. As such, social learning theory (SLT) has provided the strongest explanatory framework for the acquisition of health behaviors and interpretation of personal and environmental determinants of behaviors in children. SLT is a comprehensive theory of human behavior based on interrelations between behavioral, cognitive, and emotional processing within the individual and the surrounding physical and social environments. Congruent with motivational, self-change, and social learning theories, the intervention was designed to impart knowledge (a prerequisite to change), skills (a mechanism for change), and practice (to facilitate change), while affecting behavioral change through the child's developing abilities to self-regulate.

Program design

The intervention program was designed for small groups of four to six children, facilitated by several trained research staff. With the support and assistance of after-school program directors and childcare providers, children were recruited from after-school programs from urban, rural, and suburban communities in northern California. Composed of four 1-hour weekly sessions, the program was held at the after-school centers from which the children were recruited. Because the program required minimal supplies (a laptop computer, some small props, and a series of workbook handouts), it could be conducted in any on-site room equipped with an electrical outlet and children's furnishings, such as a classroom.

The program used motivating strategies that are appealing to children, such as a peer playgroup composed of role play activities, games, and children's media clips. Activities focused on instructing, developing, and practicing critical viewing skills; alternative choices to the target behavior (television viewing); and problem-solving strategies (Table 1). Based on theories of perceived control and motivation, the workshop activities provided the child with psychologic engagement and incentives. In effect, the children were shown how effort could be shaped and directed to produce desired outcomes. These "performance enactments" (experiences of control) help to establish behavioral change by means of the child's competence system.

The program was composed of four weekly curriculum segments. The thematic concept of each week moved from the general to the specific, focusing on knowledge and awareness, the acquisition of new skills and behaviors, and then the supportive practice and application of the skills. This natural progression of knowledge and skills development paralleled the growth and development of the children's play group. Hence, a naturally evolving group structure and dynamic were facilitated to provide increasing support for

Table 1
Intervention program

	Week 1: choices in activities	Week 2: consumerism and unhealthy foods	Week 3: risk taking/ consequences (self)	Week 4: risk taking/ consequences (others)
Curriculum concept				
Behavioral domain	Coping, motivation	Cognitive appraisal	Self-regulation	Competency (self-efficacy)
Role play	Reporters!	Detectives!	Doctors and nurses!	Coaches!
Mode	Role play of children being interviewed by a reporter regarding television viewing and alternate activities	Laptop video clip of taste tests of three different cola brands and understanding brands	Laptop video clip of action and adventure scenes with potential injuries	Laptop video clips of superheroes and conflict scenes
Group activity	Group dialog regarding such things as children's media use and favorite shows, fun activity worksheets	Cola challenge	"Emergency!" game	Group dialog of consequences and alternative problem-solving strategies
Practice	Determining children's media and lifestyle habits, motivation encouraging choice and healthy activities	Learning to look for clues regarding product contents and advertising	Preventing accidents, injuries, and illness	Learning and practicing problem solving strategies
Knowledge	Kids can choose healthier alternative activities to watching television	Commercials and ads are meant to sell you products and may not tell you everything you need to know to make healthy buying decisions	Media do not usually show real-life consequences of risky and unhealthy behaviors	Violence is not a viable solution to solving real-life problems, even though the media often portrays it as such

Skill			
Problem solving, applying concrete steps to solving problems using internal and external resources	Deconstructing special effects and identifying real life consequences of risky and unhealthy behaviors portrayed in the media	Critical thinking: reading food labels and deconstructing ads	Generating alternate activities using internal and external resources
Family and peer reinforcement			
Applying problem-solving strategies to real-life situations with peers and family, practicing problem-solving strategies by means of televised conflicts and generating alternate outcomes	Identifying harmful behaviors evidenced in daily media portrayals, practicing identifying harmful behaviors by determining when real-life injuries would result from televised behaviors and placing band-aids on TV kids while viewing television	Fostering critical analysis of ads through peer competitive play and conscious media disengagement, practicing media disengagement and critical viewing at home by means of "mute the commercials" activity	Practicing alternate activities and reinforcing healthy behaviors by means of journal and photography

the children throughout the program. Essential to learning and internalizing the information presented, each programmatic week allowed for repetition and practice within the group and at home. Although parents did not directly participate in the program, they did receive weekly information packets containing media and health concepts related to the content that the children received that week. The concept of each program segment was further reviewed during the following week in relation to the activities that children practiced at home and as an introduction for the related successive concept.

On approval from the University of California, San Francisco (UCSF) Committee on Human Research, parental consent and child assent were obtained with enrollment in the Kids TV Study program. Confidentiality, group rules, and general behavioral guidelines were discussed with the children. Children were told they would receive incentives (books and small surprises) each week of the program and a $20 gift certificate to Toys R Us on completion of the program; parents were given a gift certificate to a local restaurant or food market. These incentives were used because of the significant questionnaire response burden for the child and parent necessary for hypothesis testing over the 6-month longitudinal design in the intervention and control groups.

Using after-school programs and community sites made the intervention accessible to children and families, thereby increasing parents' willingness to participate and the overall study subject retention rate. Indeed, the program appreciated a 100% retention rate. Riesch and colleagues [47] report successful recruitment in vulnerable populations by attending to three major factors: (1) community involvement, (2) adherence to developmental principles, and (3) ease of participation for the families and communities. The after-school and community site coordinators' interest in the program, relationships with the families, and willingness to accommodate groups in their facilities proved to be critical in the successful enrollment of families and administration of the program. As gatekeepers for their communities, the program coordinators' support and trust facilitated the referral of families to the program.

Enrollment

The Kids TV Study program enrolled 145 children; however, 11 withdrew before participating in the program, primarily because of scheduling difficulties (day or time selected at the site conflicted with other after-school commitments) or changes in eligibility status. A total sample of 134 children (aged 8 and 9 years) and their mothers participated in this study (Anglo [n = 54], Latino [n = 57], and Other [n = 23], comprising 70 girls (52%) and 64 boys (48%). Working with 16 different after-school programs and community sites, the authors conducted a total of 34 groups, with an average group size of 4 children. Half of the sites with which the authors collaborated provided multiple (2 or more) groups to the study, and 25% of the sites provided 3 or more groups. Working from within an established community site made it possible for children to refer their peers to the program, as was often the case.

Week 1

The facilitator began the first group by describing a general and broad overview of the concepts that would be covered each week. The children were given a binder to house all the information and activities they received each week. A parody on *TV Guide*, the workbook was labeled "Kids TV Study TV GUIDE," to be kept near the television at home so that they could have access to information and alternatives to television. Serving as an "ice-breaking" role play designed to generate dialog, the group facilitator then played the role of a reporter, whereby the children were "interviewed" as experts for a pretend investigative report regarding children and television. To introduce the idea of alternatives to watching television, the children were asked what they would do if they could not watch television, which resulted in a list of healthier alternatives to television viewing. Worksheets summarizing alternative activities were given to the children as reinforcements.

The children's first activity would be to begin creating their own TV GUIDE. To reinforce children's participation in alternative activities, the children were challenged to practice one alternative activity each day for 1 week, and they were given a small disposable camera for their family or friends to "catch" them doing these acts. Also embedded in the challenge was the idea that the children would be behaving more healthfully than their family and friends and that they could "catch" them watching television. The children's pictures were developed by research staff the following week to be placed in their TV GUIDES as reminders of the healthy activities they chose to do.

Week 2

During the second week of the program, the children role-played being "detectives" looking for clues about actual product contents and common advertising strategies. The children participated in the "Cola Challenge," a game in which the kids try to determine the brand of soft drink they are sampling based on taste alone. In addition to learning the techniques of building brand loyalty, the children learned how to read labels and began to determine whether ingredients are helpful or harmful to their health. Handouts featuring tips on reading labels were given to the children to be placed in their TV GUIDE binders. The children also learned how commercials use special effects to sell products. To extend their new awareness of marketing strategies to daily life, the children were instructed to play "Mute the Commercials" at home, using their remote control mute button while watching television. The children were challenged to try to determine the product being advertised by looking for clues. This at-home activity was designed to reinforce disengagement from the media and to support the practice of critical viewing skills.

Week 3

The third week began with a review of the basic concepts of critical viewing applied to magazine ads for junk food, designer clothes, and cigarettes. After deconstructing the ads to reveal their emotional appeal, the ads were used to challenge the children to consider whether the message was real or fake or if the message could result in negative health consequences. The group discussed prevention, and how realistic viewing can play a part in preventing diseases or injuries from occurring in real life. The children then played a game called "Emergency!" in which teams of health care providers and patients view popular movie clips portraying risky behaviors and compete to determine the number of injuries that would have resulted in real life. Week 3 concludes with the children receiving a paper "TV Kid patient," pack of crayons, and band-aids to practice identifying and recording real-life injuries on their "patient" while they view television during the following week.

Week 4

During the final week of the program, the children role-played coaches, learning and practicing problem-solving techniques developed by Shure [48] that could help to prevent risk-taking behaviors within peer groups. The children viewed conflict scenes from superhero cartoons and determined the problem, consequence, and alternative solution to each conflict scene. The technique was then practiced on problems offered by the children, and each child was given a pocket-sized card listing the problem-solving steps to aid as a reminder and reinforcement.

Program evaluation

Child evaluations

Children's evaluations of the overall program, content specific to each week, and structure and function of the play group were solicited at the conclusion of the 4-week program. Of the 134 children enrolled in the program, 73% (n = 98) completed evaluations at the end. Based on their responses, 99% of the children considered the program "fun," 100% of the children thought that the program taught them new things, 96% thought they would participate in the program again if given the opportunity, and 96% would refer other children to the program. The children were split in their responses regarding the length of time the program encompassed, with 44% reporting that they thought the program should be longer and 47% thinking that the program length was just about right; only 9% thought that the program was too long. Children reported favoring week 3 of the program most (36%), followed by week 2 (25%), week 1 (22%), and, finally, week 4 (17%). When asked about the specific activities of each program week, children reported preferring content that included video clips (weeks 2, 3, and 4) and interactive games (weeks 2 and 3), consistent with their reporting of their favorite programmatic week. Children also reported positive experiences of the group format; 97% of the children perceived the kids in their group as getting along with each other, and 98% perceived the group facilitator as enjoying the group with the kids. Indeed, several children specifically reported that their most favorite aspect of the program was being in the peer group and that their least favorite part was having the program end. These results support the potential for success in replicating the intervention program approach successfully to recruit, engage, and retain Latino and Anglo children independent of the use of research-based funded incentives.

Parent evaluations

The authors received considerably fewer (40% [n = 53]) parent responses to program evaluation surveys, which may have been attributable to longitudinal subject burden questionnaire fatigue, because parents completed 16 instruments at four different time points regarding the research hypotheses being tested at much higher completion rates (80%–100%). Ninety-eight percent of the parents (n = 52) who completed the survey reported that the program was a positive experience, however. Eighty-two percent of parents indicated that their children evidenced behavioral changes as a result of the program; 86% noted attitudinal changes; 82% noted changes in their children's food intake; 82% noted purchasing changes; and 88% noted changes in television viewing. Regarding the utility of the parent information and incentives embedded within the program, 93% of the parents found the weekly information packets to be helpful; 95% reported the family gift certificate to be helpful; and 95% considered the children's books useful. Indeed, 94% of parents reported reading the children's books with their children. Based on their survey responses, parents commented that the program helped their children to read more and watch less television, think more critically about advertising and television programming, and read more food packaging. Other reported benefits were increases in the child's self esteem and an increased capacity to understand another point of view. Seventy-one percent of parents reported they would participate in a similar program in the future.

Summary

Overall, the Kids TV Study program was successful in recruiting and retaining children and providing a positive group environment conducive to

learning, and it was effective in producing some immediately observable behavioral changes. Although the program did not directly intervene with parents and the response rate to the survey was lower than desired, the parents
also reported changes in their family media habits, indicating larger systemic
changes resulting from the child's participation in the program. The children' and parents' evaluative feedback was also remarkably consistent.
The evaluative feedback provides some initial evidence that the theoretic un-
derpinnings on which the program was based were successful. Manuscripts
with empiric results related to specific hypotheses tested by the intervention
are currently under peer review.

This approach used motivating strategies that were appealing and familiar to children, such as the media clips, interactive games, and the peer
group format; most children reported learning a great deal and having
fun while in the program. Interestingly, many children also reported that
the thing he or she liked best about the program was being with peers in
the group. It might be argued that by placing children's viewing experience
in a larger social context, the children were motivated and reinforced to
change their behaviors. Because the progression of knowledge imparted
and skills practiced also paralleled the growth and development of the children's play group, this observation may be particularly true.

Compared with other intervention programs, this study was less resource-
intensive and did not require parent participation, potentially making the
program easily replicable. Unlike lengthy classroom-based curricula [49],
the four weekly 1-hour sessions could be easily accommodated in any after-school program and administered by trained staff on site. The intervention program required minimal supplies (a laptop computer, some small
props, and a series of workbook handouts) and could be conducted in an
on-site room equipped with an electrical outlet and children's furnishings,
such as a classroom. Video clips used within the program were copied on
compact disks, also making them easy to reproduce and use.

The authors' program evaluation data indicate that the program was successful placed in a community-based venue and that children and parents reported attitudinal and behavioral changes through their participation in it.
Further, the program was accessible and could be easily replicated in diverse
communities, making its application and utility feasible for future programs.

Intervention 2: primary care practices

Childhood physical activity and healthy lifestyles

PA is fundamental to improving and maintaining physical and mental
health. Significant evidence demonstrates the strong positive effects of PA
on several biologic indices, cardiovascular health, and behavioral and academic outcomes [50,51]. Obese children and adolescents have been shown
to exhibit lower self-esteem, which may be partially related to body

dissatisfaction or teasing by peers [52–55]. In addition, obesity has been correlated with lower health-related quality-of-life ratings, decreased physical functioning, and effects on parental emotional well-being [56]. PA in adolescents may improve their physical self-concept, a characteristic that can improve motivation for sustainable change and possibly mediate unhealthy behaviors [57,58]. Current guidelines from several national health organizations therefore recommend that children and adolescents get at least 60 minutes of cumulative activity per day and limit screen time to less than 2 hours per day [50,59–61]. The 2005 YRBS revealed that only 36% of adolescents engaged in at least 60 minutes of activity on at least 5 of the 7 preceding days, however [4].

Although most recent research has examined programs based in the school setting to increase PA among youth, the primary care clinician's office has been somewhat neglected as an important venue of influence in this area. Over recent years, the primary care health setting has transitioned more than ever before from a disease management model to one of health promotion and disease prevention. In this contemporary approach to primary care, health care providers discuss lifestyle behaviors with children and their families, and thus provide the education and support necessary to make and sustain healthy choices. Given the frequent visits that families make to the primary care office for health maintenance during childhood, an intervention toward the promotion of PA in this type of setting seems ideal.

Needs assessment

Valencia Health Services (VHS) is an integrated service-teaching practice owned and operated by the UCSF, under the direction of the Department of Family Health Care Nursing and in partnership with the San Francisco State University (SFSU) School of Nursing. VHS is a primary care provider for children in the Mission, South of Market, and Bayview-Hunter's Point districts of San Francisco, California. In 2004, 49.7% of the children and adolescents seen at VHS were Latino, 21.9% were African American, 8.9% were Asian or Pacific Islander, 7.96% were white, and 11.5% identified themselves as "other." Approximately 35% of these children had private health insurance, whereas the remainder had Medicaid, State Children's Health Insurance Program (SCHIP), or were uninsured.

Over the past few years, VHS has been tracking the BMI of its patients older than 2 years of age in addition to certain behaviors that may contribute to increased BMI. Current data show that 31.1% of children attending the VHS aged 4 to 11 years and 36.3% of teens aged 12 to 19 years have a BMI greater than 95%, which is far greater than the national average. In addition, at VHS, as many as 34.9% of the teens report never or rarely getting vigorous exercise, and 45.1% of children aged 4 to 11 years and 68.2% of teens aged 12 to 19 years are spending more than 2 hours per day on screen time.

In a recent review of PA intervention research, Estabrooks and Glasgow [62] report that despite wide dissemination of findings and guidelines for PA, weight management, and cardiovascular fitness, there is little evidence that clinical PA interventions are being translated into practice. The concerning findings from the VHS clinic prompted the design of a new approach to the promotion of PA among children and families by the authors, using a systems and relationship model of translation.

Behavioral counseling in the promotion of physical activity

There is strong evidence to support the use of behavioral counseling in conjunction with dietary monitoring, parenting skill development, and PA for the prevention of childhood overweight [29,30,63]. Creating sustainable behavior change is partially related to building intrinsic motivation for maintaining the desired behavior [64–67]. In addition, children and families make more effective and lasting behavior changes if they have more autonomy and control in managing the change process, especially if they receive support and empathy while doing so [64–68]. Although the motivation for change process is patient centered, the guidance and support of health care professionals are essential to its success.

In a survey of VHS providers, all thought that most children seen at the clinic would benefit from PA and nutrition advice and all attempted to address these issues. Nevertheless, most thought that they lacked sufficient time and resources to address these issues comprehensively. In fact, research has shown that the amount of pediatricians' and pediatric nurse practitioners' time spent on PA promotion is generally low [69–71]. Primary care providers often cite lack of time or decreased confidence as a reason for neglecting preventive counseling [72–78]. Lack of reimbursement has also been cited in explaining the low prevalence of counseling efforts among pediatricians and pediatric nurse practitioners [72,74,75,77].

Parenting skills

In a review of scientific evidence by the American Dietetic Association (ADA) [29], multidimensional family-based interventions were strongly recommended for reducing childhood overweight, specifically those including parent training. In general, parents are considered strong role models for PA and healthy behaviors, and inactivity and obesity in parents are often a problem for their children as well [79–82]. Studies of multiethnic low-income children have demonstrated that support and encouragement from their parents alone result in an increase in PA levels [83–85]. VHS providers report that a considerable number of children with borderline blood pressure, lipids, or blood sugar also had significant behavioral issues, challenging their parents' abilities to institute healthy lifestyle changes. Addressing parental misperceptions with regard to their children's health risks is also significant to promoting change. In a survey of African-American caregivers of 5- to 10-year-olds, only 44% perceived their child to have a weight problem, despite the fact that 70% of the children sampled were obese [86].

Theoretic model

Motivational interviewing (MI) is a behavioral counseling technique that has been used by health care professionals to assist patients who seek to modify unhealthy lifestyles. Motivational interviewing is a "client-centered, directive method for enhancing intrinsic motivation to change by exploring and resolving ambivalence [87]." MI guides a patient through the process of reconciling feelings of ambivalence for change with overall goals for a desired behavior [64]. Through nonjudgmental support and empathy, the counselor helps the patient and family to develop and achieve set goals while fostering confidence and autonomy. Although more research on the efficacy of MI has been done in adult populations, there is ample evidence of its effectiveness in adolescents, especially for behaviors related to substance abuse and dietary control [88,89]. Empiric support for the application of MI to the modification of parental preventive care behaviors is also increasing [88]. MI has been successfully applied to the health care setting in recent years, and evidence supports the training of health care providers in this technique [68,89,90].

Providers at VHS recognized that patient and parent readiness for change was a key factor in the success of any intervention. Velicer and colleagues [91] have proposed a transtheoretic model for a variety of types of behavioral change in adults and children. Their model has five stages: precontemplation, contemplation, preparation, action, and maintenance. Individuals in the precontemplation stage are not thinking about making a change in behavior. In the contemplation stage individuals are seriously thinking about behavior change. The preparation stage involves an attempt to stop previous behavior and an initiation of new behaviors. The action stage is a continuous period of behavioral change and maintenance, immediately following action and lasting until the problem behavior is extinguished. These stages of change are ideally suited to guide clinicians in determining a patient's and family's readiness to address changes in PA and nutrition behaviors.

Program design

Allied health professionals to support physical activity counseling

Evidence-based analysis of the literature demonstrates that multidimensional family-based programs, including behavioral and dietary counseling, parent training, nutrition education, and promotion of PA, are the most effective for overweight treatment [29,63]. In addition, it has been found that counseling by allied health professionals, as an adjunct to a provider or alone, actually produced better long-term results [92]. The use of provider support staff in obesity and PA interventions provides complimentary reinforcement for effecting sustainable behavior change and addresses barriers, such as time and reimbursement issues, that limit primary care providers. In fact, many reimbursement codes associated with nutrition and exercise counseling are only applicable to nonphysician providers [93].

Based on preliminary successful reports in Canada [94], which integrated a physical activity counselor (PAC) into the adult primary health care team, the authors' adapted their approach for the VHS nurse-managed center. During the primary care visit and using MI in addition to provider and patient design, a specific stage-based plan for increased PA was developed. The patient is referred to an allied health professional (eg, PAC) to reinforce the counseling done by the provider [92,94]. The provider uses credibility and a relationship with a patient to recommend the PA behavior change, and the PAC then provides the specialized counseling necessary to achieve this goal [92]. Fitness instructors, exercise specialists, or other individuals with experience in kinesiology or related fields are qualified to be a PAC. A PAC can provide more time interacting with a patient, has the education to counsel a family about PA and other behavior changes, and knows PA-related information in the community that may be beneficial to patients [92]. This approach avails greater time for the child and family and more intensive and effective counseling to promote behavior change and maintenance to reduce health disparities in a diverse and at-risk community population.

Summary

An extensive body of literature provides strong evidence for the substantial benefits of regular PA, decreased sedentary behaviors, and health dietary practices for multicultural children and youth. Lack of PA and poor nutrition are clearly associated with health disparity–related chronic disease onset and shortened life expectancy among ethnically diverse and multicultural individuals. A new model of pediatric primary care that gives children and families easy access to services, is culturally sensitive, and uses an innovative multidimensional team approach that maximizes provider skills and services must be implemented and evaluated.

Overall summary

Translating research findings on healthy lifestyles for children and families is not a radical or even new concept. Historically, nursing has always supported health promotion. However, until recently, the field labored under the heavy mantle of dyadic patient education without much attention to behavioral change psychology or even health literacy. Attention to development-friendly alternatives in low-demand settings for diverse communities is one step in not only thinking outside the proverbial box but in actually delivering it.

References

[1] Dryfoos JG. The prevalence of problem behaviors: implications for programs. In: Weissberg RP, editor. Enhancing children's wellness. Thousand Oaks (CA): Sage Publications; 1997. p. 17–46.
[2] Centers for Disease Control and Prevention. WISQARS leading causes of death reports, 1999–2004. National Center for Injury Prevention and Control Web site. July 10, 2007. Available at: http://webappa.cdc.gov/sasweb/ncipc/leadcaus10.html. Accessed December 2, 2007.
[3] Ogden C, Carroll M, Curtin L, et al. Prevalence of overweight and obesity in the United States, 1999–2004. JAMA 2006;295(13):1549–55.
[4] Centers for Disease Control and Prevention. Youth risk behavior surveillance—United States, 2005. MMWR Morb Mortal Wkly Rep 2006;55(SS-5):23.
[5] US Census Bureau. Selected age groups for the population by race and Hispanic origin for the United States: July 1, 2005. Press release: nation's population one third minority (Table 3). May 10, 2006. Available at: http://www.census.gov/Press-Release/www/2006/nationalracetable3.pdf. Accessed December 2, 2007.
[6] US Census Bureau. The living arrangements of children in 2005. Population profile of the United States: dynamic version. July 2007. Available at: http://www.census.gov/population/pop-profile/dynamic/LivArrChildren.pdf. Accessed December 2, 2007.
[7] DeNavas-Walt C, Proctor BD, Smith J. Income, poverty, and health insurance coverage in the United States: 2006. U.S. Census Bureau, Current Population Reports. Washington, DC: US Government Printing Office; 2007. p. 60–233.
[8] National Institutes of Health. Re-engineering the clinical research enterprise: translational research. NIH roadmap for medical research Web site. 2007. Available at: http://www.nihroadmap.nih.gov/clinicalresearch/overview-translational.asp. Accessed January 11, 2008.
[9] US Department of Health and Human Services. Healthy people 2010. Washington, DC: US Government Printing Office; 2000.
[10] Villani S. Impact of media on children and adolescents: a 10-year review of the research. J Am Acad Child Adolesc Psychiatry 2001;40(4):392–401.
[11] Polce-Lynch M, Myers BJ, Kliewer W, et al. Adolescent self-esteem and gender: exploring relations to sexual harassment, body image, media influence, and emotional expression. J Youth Adolesc 2001;30(2):225–44.
[12] Committee on Public Education. Sexuality, contraception, and the media. Pediatrics 2001; 107(1):191–4.
[13] Gerbner G. Mixed messages: television and public perceptions of medicine. Presented at: American Medical Association. Los Angeles (CA), February 5, 1987.
[14] Dietz WH. The role of lifestyle in health: the epidemiology and consequences of inactivity. Proc Nutr Soc 1996;55(3):829–40.
[15] Dietz WH, Gortmaker SL. Do we fatten our children at the television set? Obesity and television viewing in children and adolescents. Pediatrics 1985;75(5):807–12.
[16] Ekelund U, Brage S, Froberg K, et al. TV viewing and physical activity are independently associated with metabolic risk in children: the European Youth Heart Study. PLoS Med 2006;3(12):2449–57.
[17] Must A, Bandini LG, Tybor DJ, et al. Activity, inactivity, and screen time in relation to weight and fatness over adolescence in girls. Obesity (Silver Spring) 2007;15(7):1774–81.

[18] Robinson TN. Reducing children's television viewing to prevent obesity: a randomized controlled trial. JAMA 1999;282(16):1561–7.

[19] te Velde SJ, De Bourdeaudhuij I, Thorsdottir I, et al. Patterns in sedentary and exercise behaviors and associations with overweight in 9–14-year-old boys and girls—a cross-sectional study. BMC Public Health 2007;7:16.

[20] Davison KK, Marshall SJ, Birch LL. Cross-sectional and longitudinal associations between TV viewing and girls' body mass index, overweight status, and percentage of body fat. J Pediatr 2006;149:32–7.

[21] Epstein LH, Paluch RA, Gordy CC, et al. Decreasing sedentary behaviors in treating pediatric obesity. Arch Pediatr Adolesc Med 2000;154(3):220–6.

[22] Ford BS, McDonald TE, Owens AS, et al. Primary care interventions to reduce television viewing in African-American children. Am J Prev Med 2002;22(2):106–9.

[23] Lumeng JC, Appuglies D, Cabral HJ, et al. Neighborhood safety and overweight status in children. Arch Pediatr Adolesc Med 2006;160(1):25–31.

[24] Salmon J, Ball K, Crawford D, et al. Reducing sedentary behaviour and increasing physical activity among 10-year-old children: overview and process evaluation of the "Switch-Play" intervention. Health Promot Int 2005;20(1):7–17.

[25] Treuth M, Hou N, Young D, et al. Accelerometry-measured activity or sedentary time and overweight in rural boys and girls. Obes Res 2005;13(9):1606–14.

[26] Viner R, Cole T. Television viewing in early childhood predicts adult body mass index. J Pediatr 2005;147:429–35.

[27] Wiecha JL, Peterson KE, Ludwig DS, et al. When children eat what they watch. Arch Pediatr Adolesc Med 2006;160(4):436–42.

[28] Motl R, Dishman R, Saunders R, et al. Perceptions of physical and social environment variables and self-efficacy as correlates of self-reported physical activity among adolescent girls. J Pediatr Psychol 2007;32(1):6–12.

[29] American Dietetic Association. Individual-, family-, school-, and community-based interventions for pediatric overweight. J Am Diet Assoc 2006;106:925–45.

[30] Kirk S, Scott BJ, Daniels SR. Pediatric obesity epidemic: treatment options. J Am Diet Assoc 2005;105:S44–51.

[31] Peterson L, Bartelstone J, Kern T, et al. Parents' socialization of children's injury prevention: description and some initial parameters. Child Dev 1995;66:224–35.

[32] Tinsley BJ. Multiple influences on the acquisition and socialization of children's health attitudes and behavior: an integrative review. Child Dev 1992;63(5):1043–69.

[33] Sharrer VW, Ryan-Wenger NM. A longitudinal study of age and gender differences of stressors and coping strategies in school-aged children. J Pediatr Health Care 1995;9(3):123–30.

[34] Kennedy CM, Strzempko F, Danford C, et al. Children's perceptions of TV and health behavior effects. J Nurs Scholarsh 2002;34(3):289–94.

[35] Gentile DA, Walsh DA. MediaQuotient®: national survey of family media habits, knowledge, and attitudes. Minneapolis (MN): National Institute on Media and the Family; 1999.

[36] Jason LA. Self-monitoring in reducing children's excessive television monitoring. Psychol Rep 1983;53(3 Pt 2):1280.

[37] Jason LA, Rooney-Rebeck P. Reducing excessive television viewing. Child and Family Behavior Therapy 1984;6(2):61–9.

[38] Jason LA. Using a token-actuated timer to reduce television viewing. J Appl Behav Anal 1985;18(3):269–72.

[39] Jason LA, Johnson SZ, Jurs A. Reducing children's television viewing with an inexpensive lock. Child & Family Behavior Therapy 1993;15(3):45–54.

[40] Jason LA, Johnson SZ. Reducing excessive television viewing while increasing physical activity. Child & Family Behavior Therapy 1995;17(2):35–45.

[41] Singer DG, Singer JL, Zuckerman DM. Teaching television: how to use TV to your child's advantage. New York: Dial Press; 1981.

[42] Dorr A, Graves SB, Phelps E. Television literacy for young children Summer. J Commun 1980;30:71–83.
[43] Dorr A, Kovaric P, Doubleday C. Parent-child coviewing of television. Journal of Broadcasting & Electronic Media 1989;33(1):35–51.
[44] Dorr A, Rabin BE. Parents, children, and television England. Bornstein MH, editor. Applied and practical parenting. Handbook of parenting, vol. 4. Hillsdale (NJ): Lawrence Erlbaum Associates, Inc.; 1995. p. 323–51.
[45] Deci EL. The psychology of self-determination. Lexington (MA): Lexington Books; 1980.
[46] Cox CL, Miller EH, Mull CS. Motivation in health behavior: measurement, antecedents, and correlates. ANS Adv Nurs Sci 1987;9(4):1–15.
[47] Riesch SK, Tosi CB, Thurston CA. Accessing young adolescents and their families for research. J Nurs Scholarsh 1999;31(4):323–6.
[48] Shure MB, et al. I can problem solve (ICPS): an interpersonal cognitive problem solving program for children. Residential Treatment for Children and Youth 2001;18:3–14.
[49] Robinson TN, Saphir MN, Kraemer HC, et al. Effects of reducing television viewing on children's requests for toys: a randomized controlled trial. J Dev Behav Pediatr 2001;22(3): 179–84.
[50] Strong WB, Malina RM, Blimkie CJ, et al. Evidence based physical activity for school-age youth. J Pediatr 2005;146:732–7.
[51] World Health Organization. Global strategy on diet, physical activity, and health. Geneva (Switzerland): WHO; 2004.
[52] Eisenberg ME, Neumark-Sztainer D, Story M. Associations of weight-based teasing and emotional well-being among adolescents. Arch Pediatr Adolesc Med 2003;157: 733–8.
[53] Eisenberg ME, Neumark-Sztainer D, Haines J, et al. Weight-teasing and emotional well-being in adolescents: longitudinal findings from Project EAT. J Adolesc Health 2006;38: 675–83.
[54] Hesketh K, Wake M, Waters E. Body mass index and parent-reported self-esteem in elementary school children: evidence for a causal relationship. Int J Obes 2004;28:1233–7.
[55] Werrij MQ, Mulkens S, Hospers HJ, et al. Overweight and obesity: the significance of a depressed mood. Patient Educ Couns 2006;62:126–31.
[56] Friedlander SL, Larkin EK, Rosen CL, et al. Decreased quality of life associated with obesity in school-aged children. Arch Pediatr Adolesc Med 2003;157:1206–11.
[57] Dishman RK, Hales DP, Pfeiffer KA, et al. Physical self-concept and self-esteem mediate cross-sectional relations of physical activity and sport participation with depression symptoms among adolescent girls. Health Psychol 2006;25(3):396–407.
[58] Rodriguez D, Audrain-McGovern J. Physical activity, global physical self-concept, and adolescent smoking. Ann Behav Med 2005;30(3):251–9.
[59] Council on Sports Medicine and Fitness and Council on School Health. Active healthy living: prevention of childhood obesity through increased physical activity. Pediatrics 2006; 117(5):1834–42.
[60] National Association of Pediatric Nurse Practitioners. Healthy Eating and Activity Together (HEAT SM) clinical practice guideline: identifying and preventing overweight in childhood. Cherry Hill (NJ): NAPNAP; 2006.
[61] Turbett P. Position statement on exercise and physical activity. J Pediatr Nurs 2006;21(1): 80–3.
[62] Estabrooks PA, Glasgow RE. Translating effective clinic based physical activity interventions into practice. Am J Prev Med 2006;31:S45–56.
[63] Shaw K, O'Rourke P, Del Mar C, et al. Psychological interventions for overweight or obesity. Cochrane Database Syst Rev 2005;(2) CD003818.
[64] Markland D, Ryan RM, Tobin VJ, et al. Motivational interviewing and self-determination theory. J Soc Clin Psychol 2005;24(6):811–31.

[65] Matsumoto H, Takenaka K. Motivational profiles and stages of exercise behavior change. International Journal of Sport and Health Science 2004;2:89–96.

[66] Ryan RM, Deci EL. Self-determination theory and the facilitation of intrinsic motivation, social development, and well-being. Am Psychol 2000;55(1):68–78.

[67] Vansteenkiste M, Sheldon KM. There's nothing more practical than a good theory: integrating motivational interviewing and self-determination theory. Br J Clin Psychol 2006;45: 63–82.

[68] Britt E, Hudson SM, Blampied NM. Motivational interviewing in health settings: a review. Patient Educ Couns 2004;53:147–55.

[69] Galuska DA, Will JC, Serdula MK, et al. Are health care professionals advising obese patients to lose weight? JAMA 1999;282(16):1576–8.

[70] O'Brien SH, Holubkov R, Reis EC. Identification, evaluation, and management of obesity in an academic primary care center. Pediatrics 2004;114:154–9.

[71] Wee CC, McCarthy EP, Davis RB, et al. Physician counseling about exercise. JAMA 1999; 282(16):1583–8.

[72] Barlow SE, Dietz WH. Management of child and adolescent obesity: summary and recommendations based on reports from pediatricians, pediatric nurse practitioners, and registered dieticians. Pediatrics 2002;110:236–8.

[73] Cheng TL, DeWitt TG, Savageau JA, et al. Determinants of counseling in primary care pediatric practice. Arch Pediatr Adolesc Med 1999;153:629–35.

[74] Larsen L, Mandleco B, Williams M, et al. Childhood obesity: prevention practices of nurse practitioners. J Am Acad Nurse Pract 2006;18:70–9.

[75] Perrin EM, Flower KB, Garrett J, et al. Preventing and treating obesity: pediatricians' self-efficacy, barriers, resources, and advocacy. Ambul Pediatr 2005;5:150–6.

[76] Pinto BM, Goldstein MG, Marcus BH. Activity counseling by primary care physicians. Prev Med 1998;27:506–13.

[77] Story MT, Neumark-Stzainer DR, Sherwood NE, et al. Management of child and adolescent obesity: attitudes, barriers, skills, and training needs among health care professionals. Pediatrics 2002;110:210–4.

[78] Wee CC. Physical activity counseling in primary care: the challenge of effecting behavioral change. JAMA 2001;286(6):717–9.

[79] Borra ST, Kelly L, Shirreffs MB, et al. Developing health messages: qualitative studies with children, parents, and teachers help identify communications opportunities for healthful lifestyles and the prevention of obesity. J Am Diet Assoc 2003;103(6):721–8.

[80] Conner JM. Physical activity and well-being. In Bornstein MH, Corey LD, Keyes LM, The Center for Child Well-Being, et al, editors. Well-being: positive development across the life course. Mahway (NJ): Lawrence Erlbaum Associates; 2003.

[81] Fogelholm M, Nuutinen O, Pasanen M, et al. Parent-child relationship of physical activity patterns and obesity. Int J Obes Relat Metab Disord 1999;23(12):1262–8.

[82] Moag-Stahlberg A, Miles A, Marcello M. What kids say they do and what parents think kids are doing: the ADAF/Knowledge Networks 2003 family nutrition and physical activity study. J Am Diet Assoc 2003;103(11):1541–6.

[83] Klesges RC, Malott JM, Boschee PF, et al. The effects of parental influences on children's food intake, physical activity, and relative weight. Int J Eat Disord 1986;5(2):335–46.

[84] McGuire MT, Hannan PJ, Neumark-Sztainer D, et al. Parental correlates of physical activity in a racially/ethnically diverse adolescent sample. J Adolesc Health 2002;30(4):253–61.

[85] O'Loughlin J, Paradis G, Kishchuk N, et al. Prevalence and correlates of physical activity behaviors among elementary schoolchildren in multiethnic, low income, inner-city neighborhoods in Montreal, Canada. Ann Epidemiol 1999;9(7):397–407.

[86] Young-Hyman D, Herman LJ, Scott DL, et al. Care giver perception of children's obesity-related health risk: a study of African American families. Obes Res 2000;8(3):241–8.

[87] Miller WR, Rollnick S. Motivational interviewing: preparing people for change. New York: Guilford Press; 2002. p. 25.

[88] Erickson SJ, Gerstle M, Feldstein SW. Brief interventions and motivational interviewing with children, adolescents, and their parents in pediatric health care settings. Arch Pediatr Adolesc Med 2005;159:1173–80.

[89] Sindelar HA, Abrantes AM, Hart C, et al. Motivational interviewing in pediatric practice. Curr Probl in Pediatr Adolesc Health Care 2004;34:322–39.

[90] Scales R, Miller JH. Motivational techniques for improving compliance with an exercise program: skills for primary care clinicians. Curr Sports Med Rep 2003;2(3):166–72.

[91] Velicer WF, Hughes SL, Fava JL, et al. An empirical typology of subjects within stage of change. Addict Behav 1995;20:299–320.

[92] Tulloch H, Fortier M, Hogg W. Physical activity counseling in primary care: who has and who should be counseling? Patient Educ Couns 2006;64(1–3):6–20.

[93] American Academy of Pediatrics. Obesity and related co-morbidities coding fact sheet for primary care pediatricians. American Academy of Pediatrics Web site. July 2005. Available at: http://www.aap.org/obesity/Obesity%20CodingFactSheetAugust07.pdf. Accessed July 13, 2006.

[94] Fortier M, Hons WH. Project summary. The PAC project Web site. Feb 24, 2006. Available at: http://www.health.uottawa.ca/pac/index.php?page=accueil&;lang=an. Accessed July 18, 2006.

ELSEVIER
SAUNDERS

Nurs Clin N Am 43 (2008) 419–435

NURSING
CLINICS
OF NORTH AMERICA

Facilitators and Barriers for Implementing Home Visit Interventions to Address Intimate Partner Violence: Town and Gown Partnerships

Tonya Eddy, MS(N), RN[a],
Erin Kilburn, MS(N), RN[b],
Chiunghsin Chang, MS[c],
Linda Bullock, PhD, RN, FAAN[d,*],
Phyllis Sharps, PhD, RN, CNE, FAAN[e]

[a]Sinclair School of Nursing, S450, University of Missouri–Columbia,
Columbia, MO 65211, USA
[b]Sinclair School of Nursing, S405, University of Missouri–Columbia,
Columbia, MO 65211, USA
[c]Human Development and Family Studies, University of Missouri–Columbia,
314 Gentry Hall, Columbia, MO 65211, USA
[d]Sinclair School of Nursing, S327, University of Missouri–Columbia,
Columbia, MO 65211, USA
[e]Department of Community-Public Health, School of Nursing, Johns Hopkins University
525 North Wolfe Street, Room 433, Baltimore, MD 21205, USA

It has been estimated that nearly 5.3 million incidents of intimate partner violence (IPV) occur every year in the United States to women aged 18 years and older, resulting in nearly 2 million injuries and 1300 deaths [1]. IPV has been linked with immediate and long-term health, social, and economic consequences. Immediate health consequences that women experience range from minor injuries to major long-term injuries, in addition to psychologic or emotional problems, suicidal behavior, and even death [1]. These women

This work was supported by grant NR009093, "Domestic Violence Home Visitation," from the National Institute of Nursing Research. The content is solely the responsibility of the authors and does not necessarily represent the official views of the National Institute of Nursing Research or the National Institutes of Health.

* Corresponding author.
E-mail address: bullockl@missouri.edu (L. Bullock).

have also been shown to have a higher incidence of engaging in alcohol, tobacco, and substance use and abuse; unhealthy dietary behaviors, such as fasting, vomiting, and overeating; and overuse of health services [1].

Social consequences of IPV can include women being isolated from their social networks and restricted from access to services because of controlling behavior and restriction of activities by the abusive partner. In the United States, the economic impact of IPV costs billions of dollars every year in direct costs for medical and mental health care and in indirect costs related to lost productivity and death [2]. Research has also identified that women experiencing IPV are more likely to be unemployed and receiving public assistance [3].

Research examining rates of abuse in rural areas is comparable to rates present in the general population [4]. Rural women may be at an even higher risk for disparities in health care, however, not only from the abuse but from other barriers that exist unique to their living situation and environment. These barriers—poverty, underinsurance or lack of health insurance, lack of public transportation, fewer health care providers, lack of childcare, communication difficulties, and decreased job and advanced education opportunities—ultimately have an impact on their access to care [5].

Geographic isolation often makes it difficult for rural women experiencing IPV to leave and get help and for law enforcement agencies to respond [6–8]. When a woman does find a way to leave, her choices are often limited and the choice to go to a shelter may require going to an unfamiliar and often frightening urban setting. Otherwise, she may remain in the community in which the care providers and consumers know one another, making the fear of lack of anonymity a barrier to her decision on leaving [6]. Women and children who are geographically isolated and within a patriarchal social structure contribute to a social context that perpetuates male violence and social control of women [9,10].

To address health disparities within vulnerable populations, university (gown) and community (town) partnerships have been successfully used [11–14]. A university, particularly a land-grant institution, has a commitment to service within the community. In addition, the National Institutes of Health (NIH) [15] has established a roadmap to guide research initiatives from bench to practice. Town and gown partnerships help to drive research progress toward practice at a faster pace. The use of interdisciplinary partnerships and public-private partnership collaborations increases the implementation of available resources from all members of the collaboration.

Working collaboratively, with the commitment to improve health, town and gown partnerships provide a mechanism through which knowledge can flow in both directions, resulting in improved health outcomes. These partnerships empower the community members with new resources and knowledge and assist in future action planning and social change [11,13,14,16,17]. In exchange, the communities can provide university members with knowledge about the community that can help university partners to target their efforts in minimizing disparities [11,12,16,17]. The purpose of this article is to describe one town and gown partnership established to address the health disparities of women experiencing IPV and the children who are exposed to that violence. A focus group study was conducted to identify the barriers faced by the town partners as they work with victims of IPV. Findings from this study are crucial to overcome issues that home visitors (HVs) face when working with this vulnerable population of women and children.

The domestic violence enhanced home visitation story

All research has an underlying story. The Domestic Violence Enhanced Home Visitation (DOVE) research study began, as many do, with a question. If two research-based interventions known to improve pregnancy outcomes—home visitations [18–21] and an evidence-based structured IPV intervention [22]—were combined, would there be a reduction in maternal exposure to IPV, and thus decreased infant exposure to IPV, and an improvement in infant health and developmental outcomes?

Early home visitation has been an essential strategy in community health practice that has been shown to improve the health and outcomes of families and to prevent child maltreatment [19,23]. Research has shown that mothers who were visited by nurse-family partnership (NFP) nurses were less likely to be reported for child abuse [18,24]. Even without systematic assessment and intervention, nurses who visited families in their homes reported significantly less IPV after 4 years [21]. The DOVE study builds on these findings by adding a structured nurse home visitation intervention for IPV.

Using Parker and colleagues' [22] evidence-based IPV empowerment intervention, the DOVE study provides prenatal visitors (town partners) with a research-driven strategy (gown intervention) to use with pregnant women in their caseloads who are experiencing current IPV. This intervention includes a structured brochure with information addressing the cycle of violence, risk factors associated with increased risk for homicide, options available to the woman, safety planning, and IPV resources specific to their locale in addition to national hotline telephone numbers [25]. For the DOVE study, the HVs are trained in the use of the brochure by the gown partners. HVs can individualize the brochure to meet each woman's special needs by allowing each woman to share her story. The brochure can then be used to focus on the areas the woman seems to have a particular need or interest in. This empowers the woman through the ability to share her story and make choices and decisions regarding the information she is most interested in [26].

The idea of using proved methods to improve outcomes for pregnant women experiencing IPV through a town and gown partnership seemed ideal. The universities participating in the grant project forged a strong partnership with the state health department at the rural site and planned to use the prenatal home visiting programs funded by the department. After receiving notification of funding, the DOVE research team (gown) began the partnership with the town partners by training the HVs from the 12 participating counties' prenatal home visitation programs in March of 2006 (Table 1 provides details of town and gown activities). HVs from these counties included registered nurses, licensed practical nurses, social workers, and lay HVs. The initial 1-day training workshop hosted by the state health department featured Dr. Jacquelyn Campbell, a leading nurse researcher in the area of IPV, who focused on the role of the HV in screening and intervening with pregnant women experiencing IPV. This workshop was attended by 75 home visitation staff, representing all participating counties in the state-funded prenatal home visitation program.

After the IPV overview training in March (2006), a series of training sessions at the various community sites were conducted by the principal investigators and consultant of the grant between March and July (2006). The purpose of these training sessions was to prepare the HVs in the research protocols pertaining to the DOVE study. Final approval of the certificate of confidentiality from the federal government was not obtained until October 2006; thus, there was a prolonged period between training and being

Table 1
Town/gown education/communication activity summary for the DOVE study

Date	Training event	N = attended
1. March 2006	4-hour IPV training	75 participants, all counties
2. June 2006	3-day training workshop for intervention counties	24 participants, all intervention counties except 1
3. December 2006–January 2007	2-hour conference call follow-up training	40 participants, all sites
4. June 2007	1-hour conference call	28 participants, all sites except Jefferson City and St. Louis
5. July 2007	2-day workshop on IPV	40 participants, all sites except Jefferson City
6. March 2006–July 2007	Site visits by DOVE nurses	25 additional site visits completed by DOVE team among all sites July 2007
7. Ongoing	Other continuing contacts	Site visits, e-mail or telephone contact two to four times per month per site
		DOVE Nest newsletter: monthly since April 2007 sent to all sites
		Literature provided by means of e-mail or mail

able to begin recruitment for the study. To refresh the HVs in the protocols and procedures of the research study, a telephone conference call was conducted. Four different days and times were offered for the HVs, and the state health department made it known that all HVs were expected to participate in at least one of the calls.

Recruitment for the study began in January 2007. All HVs were trained in accordance with the research protocol for screening and referral of women to the DOVE study. The HVs (town) screen all women in their prenatal caseload for IPV at every home visit using the Abuse Assessment Screen (AAS) [27] and the Women's Experience with Battering (WEB) [28] instruments. Women who are pregnant and screen positive for current IPV violence are asked by the HV for their written permission to forward their name and contact information to the research team (gown). The research team then contacts the woman and arranges a convenient time and place to meet to explain the study and obtain consent for participation if she agrees.

Even though the research team maintained regular contact with the HVs through a variety of methods, including telephone calls, personal contacts, e-mails, and a monthly newsletter regarding the DOVE study (see Table 1), after several months of recruitment, referrals were coming in slowly. The explanation given by the HVs for the small number of referrals was the lack of women positive for abuse within their caseload. This did not seem plausible when the research team had found rates as high as 33% current abuse when working with a similar population enrolled in a smoking cessation intervention study in the same rural areas [29]. It was hypothesized by the gown partners that the HVs were unable to screen the women or that the women were not willing to disclose the abuse to the HVs, who lived in the same rural community. Two strategies were implemented by the gown partners to counteract these problems to increase recruitment.

First, institutional review board (IRB) approval was obtained that all pregnant women (regardless of screening positive or negative for abuse) would be asked by the HV to give their written permission to have their name and contact information given to the research team. The research team would then rescreen all women referred and consented for IPV using the AAS and WEB instruments. Women who were negative for abuse would be dropped from the study, and those who were positive would continue in the study as originally planned.

Another strategy to improve overall recruitment was holding another 2-day workshop focusing on IPV. This workshop was hosted by the state health department in July 2007. The workshop was an ideal forum for the DOVE research team (gown) to interact with the HVs (town) in a structured way to tease out issues that the HVs were having in screening and intervening with women experiencing IPV. Quantitative and qualitative methods were used to gain a better understanding of the problems and successful strategies that were present among the town partners (HVs). IRB approval was obtained from the state health department IRB and from the university IRB to conduct this quality improvement evaluation. The results of the qualitative findings are presented in this article.

Methods

Sample

HVs from all 12 counties participating in the prenatal home visiting programs were invited for the first day of the workshop, focusing on general issues of screening women for IPV. Thirty-one HVs representing the 12 counties were present on the first day, and all but 1 were female. On the second day, only HVs (n = 23) from the 6 intervention counties participated in the workshop, which focused entirely on delivering the DOVE intervention to women experiencing IPV. On the first day, the HVs attending were invited to complete a questionnaire anonymously. Twenty-six HVs, (nurses, social workers, and unlicensed HVs) filled out the questionnaire. The mean age of the participants completing the survey was 46 years, and educational experience ranged from 17.4% with a high school or general equivalency diploma (GED) education to 26% with a master's degree. On the second day, the HVs from the intervention counties were also invited to participate in focus groups. (Three HVs present on day 2 were not present on the first day; thus they did not have the opportunity to participate in the survey questionnaire.) It is not known how many of the second-day participants would have been among those completing the questionnaire on the first day.

Procedure

Before the end of the first workshop day, all attendees were invited to complete an anonymous questionnaire that included basic demographic information; issues related to IPV, including personal and professional experience; and a series of questions measuring the HV's knowledge, attitudes, and beliefs regarding IPV. On the second day, attendees present were invited to participate in focus group discussions. Participants were assigned to a focus group by numbering off from one to four. Pairs of DOVE team members led four simultaneous focus groups, which included four to six HVs. Questions that were asked during the focus group discussions are listed in Box 1. No one refused to participate in the focus groups.

One DOVE team member was designated as leader of the group—asking the questions and using cues as needed that facilitated participants' discussion of their perceptions and concerns. The second DOVE team member was responsible for recording and monitoring the time, ensuring that each question would have sufficient time for discussion. Sessions were recorded and later transcribed. Descriptive content analysis of themes within each question was used to analyze the findings. Barriers and facilitators were

---

Box 1. Questions used in focus group sessions

1. "What is it like for you to work with a woman whose partner is abusive?"
2. "What strategies seem effective in breaking the silence about abuse?"
3. "What are some fears that HVs have in initiating conversations about violence?"
4. "What issues with your work can you foresee when women in your caseload participate in research studies?"

---

noted within each of the questions asked during the focus group session. Subcategories were also noted within the themes, adding depth to the data describing HV experiences working with pregnant women experiencing IPV. A coding matrix was reviewed by several DOVE team members to obtain consensus on recurrent themes.

Results

Eighty-four percent (n = 23) of the HVs participating on day 1 of the workshop completed the survey questionnaire. From the survey, the HVs' own personal experience with family violence was obtained. Table 2 presents the type of abuse experienced by the HVs. Personal experiences with physical, sexual, and emotional abuse were reported by many. Physical abuse was reported to have occurred with 16% (n = 4) of the HVs during their childhood, with 28% (n = 7) reporting having witnessed it during their childhood. Twenty-four percent of the HVs (n = 6) experienced physical abuse as adults. Sexual abuse occurred with 21% (n = 5) in childhood, with 9% (n = 2) witnessing it in childhood. As adults, 13% (n = 3) of the HVs had experienced sexual abuse. Twenty percent (n = 5) of the HVs

Table 2
Number and percent of home visitor personal experience with abuse

	Physical abuse (n = 25)	Sexual abuse (n = 23)	Emotional abuse (n = 25)	Total[a] (n = 25)
Childhood	4 (16%)	5 (21%)	5 (20%)	6 (24%)
Witnessed in childhood	7 (28%)	2 (9%)	8 (32%)	8 (32%)
Adult	6 (24%)	3 (13%)	6 (24%)	7 (28%)
No. individual women per category	8 (32%)	6 (26%)	9 (36%)	9 (36%)

[a] Questionnaires with missing data on abuse items were excluded from some analyses.

reported emotional abuse during childhood, with 32% (n = 8) having witnessed it during their childhood, and 24% (n = 6) experienced emotional abuse as adults.

The mean age of participants identified as abused (n = 9) was 45 years of age and 47 years for nonabused HVs (n = 14) (Table 3). The HVs who identified as being abused had an average of 17 years of education, whereas those nonabused had an average of 15 years. The average numbers of years working in health care for the abused and nonabused HVs were 9 and 13, respectively. On the average, HVs identified as being abused had worked 5 years with IPV and had completed five training sessions related to the issue; HVs identified as nonabused had worked an average of 3 years with IPV and had completed two training sessions.

Focus group results

A summary of barriers and facilitators to working with women who are victims of IPV as noted by the HVs during the focus group session is provided. As appropriate, supporting dialog from focus group participants is included.

Barriers

Barriers identified by HVs dealt primarily with their own emotions, which revolved around stress and frustration. They indicated that feelings of inadequacy, whether inadequacy related to assessment of their client's risk for or experience of IPV or feeling inadequately prepared to assist the client when IPV is identified, were a source of stress.

> I think that my struggle is feeling a little inadequate and not knowing what to say, I can encourage them and tell them that what is happening is not okay... I don't know the perfect thing to say, as others said taking it home and being so upset and thinking I don't know how long you can do this type of work since it affects me so much. So a variety of emotions...

Other participants noted feeling stress when the client divulged that she was a victim of IPV.

> I feel that it is stressful and challenging to find immediate resources and solutions especially if the woman cannot leave...and I feel kinda powerless and helpless.

Table 3
Descriptive information from the home visitors completing the survey

Demographics	Abused (n = 9)	Nonabused (n = 14)
Mean age	45	47
Mean years of education	17	15
Mean years in health care	9	13
Mean years working with IPV	5	3
Mean no. training sessions	5	2

Stress and frustration also occur when the HV is attempting to control her own emotions while working with the client.

> My stress comes into the point of being able to control my feelings... I wept and I felt bad about that because we are trained not to cry with the family because the concern is that you're going to make her feel bad. Which in one sense it did make her feel bad but I guess in a good sense it shows her that I am very sympathetic and that I feel her pain in some sense and I am also concerned that as I continued to work with this mom if I will be able to handle the emotional part of it.

Another identified stressful barrier is discomfort of the unknown variables in the environment. One HV described this as the following:

> I am comfortable working with the woman—uncomfortable at times in the home—but comfortable with the women. Especially the first visit, not knowing the layout, not knowing the abuser's schedule where he might be or where he might come from.

Frustration was also described by a few HVs as a barrier when working with victims of IPV. They were frustrated when their clients admitted to abuse, sometimes repeatedly, yet would not take their suggestions to increase their safety.

> ...but it becomes kinda frustrating because they repeat their story over and over and we don't seem to be getting anywhere.

Some HVs stated that their clients would show signs of abuse yet were hesitant to admit, even when confronted by the HV.

> I said that is very unusual bruising and you don't normally see bruises like that do you know how it happened? And then she said that 'No, no I don't know how I got them.' Then I described them and I put my fingers into the bruises and said that it looks like that someone really pressed their hands hard into your arm—that is what it looks like to me...

To be fair, it should be noted that some of the HVs described working with IPV victims as rewarding.

> Feeling rewarded that you were able to make a difference even if she didn't leave or do something else but giving her those options.
> ...It makes me feel good to be there and allow the mom to let her air her issues, and encourage her in any way I can, and just be a very supportive person for her because I know that most of my moms are very isolated...

Another barrier to having HVs screen for IPV involves the fears and comfort level of the HV with initiating conversations dealing with violence. HVs in the focus group session admitted to having feelings of fear associated with clients admitting violence to when they screen for violence. The fears vocalized by the HV participants included: "...making a fool of myself," fear of inability to help the client appropriately, fear of offering help that is not taken, and fear for themselves and their clients.

I think that it is just a hard topic to talk about it in general, and stumbling over my words and making a fool of myself for not knowing where to go with it in the conversation and getting lost in my words a lot of time.

I think that one of the concerns that I have seen over the years is that once the client has disclosed and you begin to talk to her about what to do whether if she feels like she is in danger or eminent danger or what. And then you offer those measures to her or those ideas and then they don't do anything. And then you feel hopeless like what do I do now because they don't want to take that.

...so you don't want to cause more harm—so you do not want to push too far—push them too much too soon and you don't want them in danger or yourself in danger.

It was obvious that the HVs are eager to assist their clients in any way necessary but are reluctant to act if they perceive their actions could potentially cause the client more harm. Not knowing about the abuse seemed to be perceived by the HV as having more freedom to assist the client with other health disparity barriers (eg, prenatal care, medical needs, environmental health). Once IPV was identified, the HV was obligated to address the issue, which was noted by them as an awkward situation, although most of the HVs agreed that it was significantly important.

Facilitators

Many of the HVs in the focus groups admitted to previously or currently having women in their caseloads who had admitted abuse. HVs with this experience were helpful in identifying methods they have used to improve communication with their clients, increasing the potential that the client is open to talking about the abuse. Admitting to the abuse allows the HV to provide the client with information, materials, and resources that may be helpful.

Building good rapport with the client was the most frequently mentioned strategy to open communication. Many HVs described stories in which clients only admitted to abuse in their relationship after many visits by the HV, sometimes after many years as their client.

You just build a trust with them. You build a friendship with them. They get to know you and you know them. And it's just going to happen over time, you may not get it the first few weeks or that first month but you are going to get it in time—that relationship.

...it just takes some time and the families I work with I get them for two years and we have a long cycle and it is going to happen again and again and so you want us to fix it now and that is not the way I look at these things. They are making some life changes and it just takes some time and trust.

Other participants note the use of voice inflection and nonverbal cues as important when working with IPV victims. Being careful not to intimidate, seem to persuade, or belittle women in their caseload helps them to gain the respect needed for women to feel comfortable in discussing difficult topics, such as abuse.

> I work with teens so I really have to watch my facial expressions and they are looking at my reaction—and so many times I have to mention it in casual conversation and usually they will respond and let me know sometimes on the first visit and sometimes a bit later.
>
> I would say that eye contact is so much. That when they start the conversation and they can't look at you directly and you show them that respect that you are listening, then by the end there is, you can tell that they are receptive.

Barriers working with gown partners

When asked about barriers noted within their own experience working with research teams, many HVs at first denied negative issues related to working with research in their job. Many noted that having a research team available was a relief and a good resource for themselves and their clients. As discussion progressed, a few participants did reveal negative issues related to having their clients in a research study.

The most common negative issue discussed by the HVs revolved around perceived interference or risk for interference by the research nurses with the carefully built relationship between the client and themselves. HVs described fear that their clients would not view their relationships in the same manner since the HVs now knew that the clients were abused.

> The only concern I have is that when I give this girl this paper and she consents for you guys to call her that she thinks back in her mind and then thinks that she shouldn't, we shouldn't visit any more. I have one girl that had consented to be called and we had a pretty good relationship with her and she was getting ready to deliver and she up and left and she didn't call me... So in the back of my mind I keep thinking that she didn't call me because I had gotten her hooked up and she hadn't told me anything before and now I knew.

One HV was concerned that research involvement and the added responsibilities of participation would overwhelm her clients at a time when they were already stressed.

> Our specific program has a lot of requirements as part of our program so we have issues with overwhelming them with too many people coming into their home...and so we are asking them to do one more thing and even though they are going to get paid, they get paid with the other things too so it is just one more requirement and it may stress them too much.

It is interesting that themes identified as negative aspects of having clients involved in research were all framed as negative for the client. No comments were noted as the involvement being negative for the HV. The only comment related to the amount of time needed for the HV to complete the DOVE intervention dealt with the time needed being an inconvenience for the client rather than for the HV.

It should be noted that previous communication from individuals at various prenatal home visiting sites indicated that one possible rationale for decreased referral rate by the HVs was the fear that DOVE team nurses would "take over" their clients' care, breaking the carefully forged relationship the HV had developed with her or his clients. No mention of this barrier was noted during the focus group sessions. Conversely, when probed regarding the topic of "feeling like the DOVE nurse would take over," focus group participants denied this fear.

Discussion

The information obtained from the HVs participating in this study provides the gown partners with valuable insights about town partners' perceptions of barriers they face when working with this particular group of vulnerable women and with the research team. Because the town partners hold the key to identifying abused women, and thus helping to eliminate the health disparities this group faces, it is crucial that the gown partners understand these barriers.

One of the main barriers regarding screening for IPV noted in the focus groups, and in numerous research studies [30–40], is related to the lack of knowledge and training that health care professionals receive: knowledge related to violence and warning signs; not knowing how to ask about violence; lack of knowledge regarding legal options and social services; and how to help in general. This lack of knowledge seemed to fuel the HVs' stress and fear of working with abused women. Numerous meetings with the HVs and various workshops regarding the DOVE study have attempted to break down this barrier by providing information and special training to allow the HVs to become more comfortable with addressing the topic of IPV. The authors' experience shows that multiple sessions are needed. Providing the opportunity for the HVs to communicate openly and honestly about their experiences and feelings of dealing with women in abusive relationships reinforces that the work they are doing is important, and the knowledge helps to alleviate some of the fear. The town and gown partnership provides the HVs with the evidence-based knowledge and hands-on experience needed to assist and empower the women they are working with to make decisions regarding their safety and that of these women's children.

Whether screening for abuse in an institutional setting or rural home visit, providers have expressed their concerns regarding inadequate knowledge about the identification and treatment of women experiencing violence and the IPV resources a provider has available to offer women identified [30,31,35,36,38,40–42]. There are unique barriers experienced by rural providers related to resources, such as law enforcement agencies slow response to reports of abuse because of the distance required to travel to the site of the violence and fewer shelters being available in rural areas [8,30,31,41,42]. Even when available, rural women are often hesitant to use the shelter in their area because of the risk for loss of anonymity. This fear can hinder a woman's decision to leave her abuser. Providers from rural and urban settings also express their concerns over offending the woman by asking about abuse. Rural providers may differ in that, many times, the provider may know the woman she is helping personally or may know her abuser. This seems to be more of a concern for rural health care providers than for those in the urban setting, in which additional resources are available to help provide the anonymity that abused women prefer [31,32,41,42].

Within hospitals and clinics, lack of time is cited as a major barrier in addition to lack of privacy for screening, fear of offending the victim or client, inconsistency in screening guidelines, cultural values and influences, lack of support, and nurses' own personal experiences with violence [39,43–47]. The HVs from the focus groups also expressed fear about offending their clients, being uncomfortable with the screening tools, not knowing what resources were available, or what to do if the woman admitted to being abused, in addition to disclosing their own personal experiences or history of violence in their lives. It was clear from the focus groups that the women's well-being was the top concern for the HVs, such that when they realized they may be further victimizing a woman by not screening, some of their own fears seemed to dissipate.

Nursing implications to screening for abuse

The personal history of abuse experienced by the HVs (see Table 2) is similar to current documented rates of abuse in the general population. Nursing care of the victims of abuse can be affected positively or negatively by health care providers' past abuse experiences. The professional role and culture of health care can help to make this care more positive than negative.

Nursing education emphasizes the importance of separating personal values, past experiences, and opinions from professional responses to clients. This neutrality is meant to avoid reacting on the basis of personal experiences and viewpoints and imposing them on others. Empathy is another characteristic of nursing education and forms the basis for a helping relationship [48]. Providing understanding and sensitivity to others' feelings, emotions, or situations may become difficult, and nurses may distance themselves when they themselves may be dealing with similar issues. It may also be to the client's benefit to receive care from nurses who have also been victims of IPV, however, because they may be even more sensitive to patients' situations. When reviewing transcripts from the focus groups and demographic survey, several HVs admitted that their own similar personal experiences influence the care they provide.

> I can say that I have had a family member that has been abused and one thing that I have seen and I know is that you can't make them get out until they are ready...that is one thing that I have seen... I have seen my mom and all kinds of family going over trying and they keep going back so it is a cycle, you can't force anyone until they are ready, you can be there and empathize with them but if they aren't ready they aren't ready.

Limitations of study and application to future practice and research

It is important to note that this study is limited in several ways. First, the sample was a convenience sample of HVs already involved in the DOVE study. Second, the focus group interviews included a time limit imposed by the workshop schedule, and there was a possibility for decreased participation related to group dynamics. In addition, although a strength of the study is the inclusion of HVs from urban, suburban, and rural areas, all participants were located in a single midwestern state, decreasing generalizability to other regions of the United States or globally.

As noted with these HVs, and as previous research has shown, many have personal and professional issues addressing IPV with their clients. Nurses who have experienced abuse may or may not be as effective in identifying and intervening with patients who are experiencing abuse. More research is needed in this area to determine what effect prior experiences have on nurses' behaviors. Providing assistance to these nurses to acknowledge their own personal emotions, values, and opinions related to their traumatic abuse may allow them to be more successful in assessing, identifying, and intervening with battered women within their individual caseloads.

The DOVE study's town and gown partnership is one example of how collaboration between researchers and health care providers in a rural setting can help each other to learn and grow while helping to strengthen and support a climate for social change. This partnership can also enhance the well-being, health, and provision of resources to this vulnerable population of women and children experiencing abuse through evidence-based interventions.

Acknowledgments

The DOVE research team includes Jacquelyn Campbell, PhD, RN, FAAN, Linda Rose, PhD, RN, Megan Bair-Merritt, MD, Kim Hill, MS, Keisha Walker, MS, RN, Alyssa McCray, BS, RN, and Etasha Crowder, BS, RN, from Johns Hopkins University School of Nursing; and Janis Davis, BS, RN, Kathleen Ellis, MS, RN, Karen Rupright, BS, RN, Karen Mickey, MS, RN, Shreya Bhandari, MS, and Katharine Ball, MS from the University of Missouri Sinclair School of Nursing.

[24] Kitzman H, Olds DL, Henderson CR, et al. Effect of prenatal and infancy home visitation pregnancy outcomes, childhood injuries and repeated childbearing: a randomized controlled trial. JAMA 1997;278:644–52.

[25] Sharps P. Domestic violence enhanced home visitation program—DOVE, National Institutes of Health/National Institutes of Nursing Research. Bethesda (MD): NIH; 2004.

[26] Dutton MA. Empowering and healing the battered woman. New York: Springer; 1992.

[27] McFarlane J, Parker B, Soeken K, et al. Assessing for abuse during pregnancy. Severity and frequency of injuries and associated entry into prenatal care. JAMA 1992;267(23): 3176–8.

[28] Coker AL, Pope BO, Smith PH, et al. Assessment of clinical partner violence screening tools. J Am Med Womens Assoc 2001;56(1):19–23.

[29] Bhandari S, et al. Comparative analyses of stressors experienced by rural low-income pregnant women experiencing intimate partner violence and those who are not. J Obstet Gynecol Neonatal Nurs 2008. (in press).

[30] Eastman BJ, Bunch SG. Providing services to survivors of domestic violence: a comparison of rural and urban service provider perceptions. J Interpers Violence 2007;22(4):465–73.

[31] Eastman BJ, Bunch SG, Williams AH, et al. Exploring the perceptions of domestic violence service providers in rural localities. Violence Against Women 2007;13:700–16.

[32] Roberts LW, Battaglia J, Epstein RS. Frontier ethics: mental health care needs and ethical dilemmas in rural communities. Psychiatr Serv 1999;50(4):497–503.

[33] Parsons LH, Zaccaro D, Wells B, et al. Methods of and attitudes toward screening obstetrics and gynecology patients for domestic violence. Am J Obstet Gynecol 1995;173: 381–6.

[34] Wright RJ, Wright RO, Isaac NE. Response to battered mothers in the pediatric emergency department: a call for an interdisciplinary approach to family violence. Pediatrics 1997; 1997(99):186–92.

[35] Waalen J, Goodwin MM, Spitz AM, et al. Screening for intimate partner violence by health care providers: barriers and interventions. Am J Prev Med 2000;19(4):230–7.

[36] Goff HW, Shelton AJ, Byrd TL, et al. Preparedness of health care practitioners to screen women for domestic violence in a border community. Health Care Women Int 2003;24: 135–48.

[37] Hinderliter D, Doughty AS, Delaney K, et al. The effect of intimate partner violence education on nurse practitioners' feelings of competence and ability to screen patients. J Nurs Educ 2003;42(10):449–54 (8 ref).

[38] Yonaka L, Yoder MK, Darrow JB, et al. Barriers to screening for domestic violence in the emergency department. J Contin Educ Nurs 2007;38(1):37–45.

[39] Gutmanis I, Beynon C, Tutty L, et al. Factors influencing identification of and response to intimate partner violence: a survey of physicians and nurses. BMC Public Health 2007;7:12. Available at: http://www.biomedcentral.com/1471-2458/7/12.

[40] Hegge M, Condon BA. Nurses' educational needs regarding battered women. J Nurs Staff Dev 1996;12(5):229–35.

[41] Control C f D. Rural health-care providers' attitudes, practices, and training experience regarding intimate partner violence—West Virginia, March 1997. MMWR Morb Mortal Wkly Rep 1998;47(32):670–3.

[42] Bosch K, Schumm WR. Accessibility to resources: helping rural women in abusive partner relationships become free from abuse. J Sex Marital Ther 2004;30:357–70.

[43] Cullinane PM, Alpert EJ, Freund KM. First-year medical students' knowledge of, attitudes toward, and personal histories of family violence. Acad Med 1997;72(1):48–50.

[44] Diaz-Olavarrieta C, Paz F, de la Cadena CG, et al. Prevalence of intimate partner abuse among nurses and nurses' aides in Mexico. Arch Med Res 2001;32:79–87.

[45] Ellis JM. Barriers to effective screening for domestic violence by registered nurses in the emergency department. Crit Care Nurs Q 1999;22(1):27–41.

References

[1] National Center for Injury Prevention and Control (NCIPC): Intimate partner vi
sheet [electronic] Atlanta GA: Centers for Disease Control and Prevention. 2005
at: http://www.cdc.gov/ncipc/factsheets/ipvfacts.htm. Accessed 10/24/2005 .

[2] Max W, Rice D, Finkelstein E, et al. The economic toll of intimate partner violen
women in the United States. Violence Vict 2004;19(3):259–72.

[3] Lloyd S, Taluc N. The effects of male violence on female employment. Violenc
Women 1999;5:370–92.

[4] Hightower NR, Gorton J. Domestic violence among patients at two rural health ca
prevalence and social correlates. Public Health Nurs 1998;15(5):355–62.

[5] Bushy A. Health issues of women in rural environments: an overview. J Am Med
Assoc 1998;53:53–6.

[6] Adler C. Unheard and unseen: rural women and domestic violence. J Nurse Midwife
41:463–6.

[7] Websdale N. Rural woman battering and the justice system: an ethnography. Th
Oaks (CA): Sage Publications; 1997.

[8] Davis K, Taylor B, Furniss D. Narrative accounts of tracking the rural domestic v
survivors' journey: a feminist approach. Health Care Women Int 2001;22:333–47.

[9] Gagne PL. Appalachian women: violence and social control. J Contemp Ethnogr 1992
387–415.

[10] Denham SA. Describing abuse of pregnant women and their healthcare workers in
Appalachia. MCN Am J Matern Child Nurs 2003;28(4):264–9.

[11] Evans GD, Rey J, Hemphill M, et al. Academic-community collaboration: an ecolog
early childhood violence prevention. Am J Prev Med 2001;20(1):22–30.

[12] Carey TS, Howard D, Goldmon M, et al. Developing effective interuniversity partner
and community based research to address health disparities. Acad Med 2005;80
1039–45.

[13] Thompson LS, Story M, Butler G. Use of a university-community collaboration mod
frame issues and set an agenda for strengthening a community. Health Promot P
2003;4(4):385–92.

[14] Williams A, Labonte R, Randall J, et al. Establishing and sustaining community-univer
partnerships: a case study of quality of life research. Crit Public Health 2005;15(3):291–3

[15] Health, N.I.H. NIH roadmap initiatives. Washington, DC: National Institute of Heal
2007.

[16] El Ansari W, Phillips CJ, Zwi AB. Narrowing the gap between academic professional w
dom and community lay knowledge: perceptions from partnerships. Public Health 200
116(3):151–9.

[17] Lomas J. Using 'linkage and exchange' to move research into policy at a Canadian founda
tion. Health Aff (Millwood) 2000;19(3):236–40.

[18] Olds DL, Eckenrode J, Henderson C, et al. Long-term effects of home visitation on materna
life course and child abuse and neglect: fifteen-year follow-up of a randomized trial. JAMA
1997;278:637–43.

[19] Olds DL, Hill P, Robinson J, et al. Update on home visiting for pregnant women and parents
of young children. Curr Probl Pediatr 2000;30:107–41.

[20] Olds DL, Kitzman H, Cole R, et al. Effects of nurse home-visiting on maternal life course and
child development: age 6 follow-up results of a randomized trial. Pediatrics 2004;114:1550–9.

[21] Olds DL, Robinson J, Pettitt L, et al. Effects of home visits by paraprofessionals and by
nurses: age 4 follow-up results of a randomized trial. Pediatrics 2004;114:1560–8.

[22] Parker B, McFarlane J, Soeken K, et al. Testing an intervention to prevent further abuse to
pregnant women. Res Nurs Health 1999;22:59–66.

[23] Chalk R, King PA. Violence in families: assessing prevention and treatment programs.
Washington, DC: National Academy Press; 1998.

[46] Moore ML, Zaccaro D. Attitudes and practices of registered nurses toward women who have experienced abuse/domestic violence. J Obstet Gynecol Neonatal Nurs 1998;27(2): 175–82.

[47] Yoshihama M, Mills LG. When is the personal professional in public child welfare practice? The influence of intimate partner violence and child abuse histories on workers in domestic violence cases. Child Abuse Negl 2003;27:319–36.

[48] Stuart GW, Laraia M. Principles and practice of psychiatric nursing. 8th edition. St. Louis (MO): Elsevier Mosby; 2005.

ELSEVIER
SAUNDERS

NURSING
CLINICS
OF NORTH AMERICA

Nurs Clin N Am 43 (2008) 437–447

African Americans with Memory Loss: Findings from a Community Clinic in Lexington, Kentucky

Deborah D. Danner, PhD[a,b,*],
Charles D. Smith, MD[a,c,d], Peace Jessa, MD[a,b],
JoAnna Hudson, RN[a]

[a]Sanders-Brown Center on Aging, Alzheimer's Disease Center, University of Kentucky,
Lexington, KY, USA
[b]Department of Preventive Medicine and Environmental Health, College of Public Health,
University of Kentucky, Lexington, KY, USA
[c]Department of Neurology, College of Medicine, University of Kentucky,
Lexington, KY, USA
[d]Magnetic Resonance Imaging Center, College of Medicine, University of Kentucky,
Lexington, KY, USA

The clinical outreach program described in this report was created to address the lack of use of dementia care services by African Americans in central Kentucky. Although not a problem unique to Kentucky, African Americans did not take advantage of dementia services offered through the University of Kentucky's (UK) Alzheimer's Disease Center (ADC), although the same services were in high demand by white members of the region.

African Americans have an increased risk for the development of Alzheimer's disease (AD) [1–5]; yet, they underuse existing dementia services and are underrepresented in dementia research, creating an alarming national trend [6,7]. Without their participation, the medical community is left without the necessary knowledge for developing effective prevention and treatment programs specific and appropriate for them. Furthermore, African-American patients who have dementia and their families struggle unnecessarily without the care and support that they need.

This work was supported in part by grant 90AZ2693 from the Administration on Aging and grant 1P30-AG0-28383 from the National Institute on Aging.

* Corresponding author. Sanders-Brown Center on Aging, Alzheimer's Disease Center, University of Kentucky, 800 South Limestone, Lexington, KY 40536–0230.

E-mail address: dddann00@uky.edu (D.D. Danner).

AD, the most common form of dementia, has assumed national visibility as a public health issue, in large part, because of the aging of the country's population. Age is the greatest risk factor for the development of AD [8]. Currently, African Americans represent the nation's largest minority group of older Americans, with African Americans aged 85 years and older being the most rapidly growing age group [9]. Increased numbers of older African Americans create increased numbers of African Americans with AD.

The risk for the development of AD symptoms is greater for African Americans than for whites, with estimates of increased risk ranging from 15% to 100% [1–5]. Multiple genetic, environmental, and social factors likely contribute to this risk. For example, African Americans have hypertension prevalence rates that are among the world's highest [10]. It is known that hypertension and elevated cholesterol may double the risk for AD [11]. Also, African Americans are 43% more likely than their white counterparts to have a biologic first-degree relative with AD [12], thus increasing their chances of developing AD because of a potential genetic predisposition. Finally, African Americans have higher rates of type II diabetes, a factor that influences the development of vascular disease and vascular dementia [13]. Brain injury attributable to vascular factors may compound AD. Dietary patterns also are implicated as contributing to disease development, with dietary habits being tied not only to cultural traditions but to economic factors [14].

Research supports the strong role of religion and family and the importance of community in the development of health care programs for African Americans [15]. African Americans prefer to care for their loved ones at home, often using extended family in a care process that is largely female dominated [15]. Research suggests that over the course of AD, African Americans receive services later than whites and sometimes do not seek medical care at all, suggesting that African Americans more frequently view AD as a normal part of the aging process and are less likely to institutionalize a loved one [16]. Dilworth-Anderson and Gibson [17] suggest that the variance in cultural beliefs about dementia contributes to various factors, including who offers care, why that person offers care, and whether or not to institutionalize. They state that, depending on the particular cultural group, the behaviors of a demented older person may not be brought to the attention of medical professionals; instead, these behaviors may be considered normal or treated at home [17].

In spite of their greater need, African Americans did not seek diagnosis, treatment, or support at the UK's ADC during its first 15 years. Slavery, segregation, and racism, blatant and subtle, had created barriers of trust between African Americans and that research center. University faculty, health care staff, and research scientists were predominantly white. Moreover, most African Americans were aware of the Tuskegee study [18], where research into the long-term effects of syphilis involved deceiving African-American participants and providing no treatment, creating a general distrust of research conducted by whites [19]. Additionally, it was not uncommon for federally subsidized health care programs to be feasibility or pilot programs, and these programs were often dropped when funding ended, creating a sense of impermanence and lack of long-term commitment to the health of African Americans.

The National Institutes of Health recognized the limitations of research that did not include a sample population representative of the general population and began requiring racial and ethnic representation in federally funded research. UK scientists at the ADC were aware of this need and made numerous unsuccessful attempts to recruit African Americans, the largest minority group in the service area, to use established dementia care programs and to participate in AD research. Despite these efforts, in 2003, only 3% of patients being evaluated at the UK-ADC memory disorders clinic were African American in an area in which African Americans constituted 13% of the local population. African-American participation in research was even lower.

Although underuse of health services and lack of representation in research by African Americans were nationwide issues, the dementia care program in Kentucky faced local barriers. Despite legislation against racial discrimination, economic factors remained, and neighborhoods in Lexington remained largely segregated by race. As a border state during the Civil War, Kentucky became a primary stop on the Underground Railroad. With emancipation, many former slaves went north for a better life, leaving behind encapsulated community enclaves that are perhaps unique to border states. In the nineteenth century, Kentucky's Berea College was open to individuals of any race until Kentucky passed the Day Law, which forbade blacks and whites from attending the same school. More recently, within living memory for many older African Americans, the first black student to attend the UK, Lyman T. Johnson, had to file a lawsuit to do so. Given this history of discrimination within the nation and the state, the UK's ADC health care providers faced serious mistrust from the African-American community.

Approach

The first step in the Kentucky plan to provide dementia care to African Americans was to place quality treatment and services in a north-side neighborhood. The authors acquired the use of examination rooms in an existing clinic run through the UK located in the Lexington neighborhood, with the highest proportion of African-American residents. They then recruited an African-American nurse from the local community to assist with clinical activities. During the first 2 years of operation, the authors found that simply opening a dedicated dementia clinic and hiring an African-American nurse were not sufficient to attract and serve those in need of care. During the first year, 20 individuals were evaluated, and in the second year, 10 individuals were evaluated. Clearly, barriers to African Americans making full use of the clinic remained.

In 2003, with 3 years of funding provided by an Administration on Aging (AOA) grant, the authors refined their approach to the development of dementia care and created the African-American Dementia Outreach Partnership (AADOP). Expanded interrelated objectives were developed to accomplish the goal of making quality dementia care available to all segments of the community. Program objectives were (1) to identify and overcome barriers that inhibited the use of available clinical and support services for patients who had dementia and their families, (2) to increase awareness of AD and foster greater understanding of the importance of research, and (3) to provide quality care that was sensitive to the unique needs and values of the African-American community.

An essential element of the expanded effort involved community collaboration. The AOA effort was designed to establish a partnership between groups and agencies with a shared commitment to providing equal health care access to African Americans with dementia. The original partnership consisted of the UK's ADC, the Commonwealth of Kentucky's Division of Aging and Independent Living, and the Greater Kentucky and Southern Indiana Chapter of the Alzheimer's Association. Representatives of the partnership met monthly to discuss program plans and activities. Decisions were made as a group.

Objective 1

To identify barriers and accomplish the AADOP's first objective, the authors turned to leaders within the African-American community and families and listened. Focus groups identified African-American attitudes and beliefs in addition to the suspected distrust of the white university culture. Barriers that were identified included a lack of awareness of the disease and confusion in those the authors sought to reach about what changes in memory were normal and what changes might indicate a medical disorder. A stigma was found to be associated with AD and other mental health problems, making families hesitant to seek help. Families thought that problems with their older relatives were personal business and their task to shoulder, and their unwavering respect for their elders made them hesitant to seek outside assistance. Many were unaware of the newly established neighborhood clinic.

The authors decided to turn to the most trusted institution in African-American families, the church, for help in reaching the target population. Six large African-American churches were identified, and contact with their senior pastors was established. After two meetings with the ministers, with one meeting providing requested information to the ministers on the latest findings on AD and its impact on the African-American community, the six churches became active members of the outreach partnership and formed an Advisory Council of Ministers to guide the program. A separate advisory council of diverse community leaders and family representatives was established and also met quarterly.

The Advisory Council of Ministers' endorsement of the AADOP did not happen at the first meeting with them. Ministers voiced concern that AADOP efforts might end when funding ended, and only when they were assured that financial arrangements had been made to continue the clinic did they begin to recognize the sincerity of the outreach for their people. Ministers also expressed their concern about working with the university and questioned the authors' motives. The authors acknowledged earlier injustices and emphasized the need for their help with this effort to improve health care for African Americans.

Objective 2

In planning educational activities so that they would successfully increase awareness of AD among the local population, the authors used findings from their own focus groups and sought input from their advisory boards. Recommendations were that the authors broaden their outreach by attending festivals and other local events targeted to older African Americans in addition to continuing presentations at churches and senior centers. It was suggested that the authors become a visible presence in the community they were serving by attending health fairs and offering free memory check-ups. The authors were told that how the message was presented was important in determining how it was received, urging them to keep it simple. For example, it was suggested that the authors talk about memory loss, a symptom that African Americans would understand immediately, rather than dementia or AD in initial publications and outreach. To ensure that the community surrounding the clinic was aware of the new memory care services, an open house to introduce the program was suggested.

Objective 3

The clinical approach was designed to minimize the amount of time the patient and family spend in a medical setting. The authors wanted the clinic to be as nonthreatening and friendly as possible. Neuropsychologic testing and the collection of standardized social and medical data took place in the patient's home and were conducted by African-American clinicians. By completing the testing in the home and having an examiner of the same race, patients were more comfortable with testing and the clinician developed a better understanding of what services might be appropriate for the family. Home evaluations allowed rapport to be established between AADOP health care professionals and families before the first clinic visit, which minimized the number of individuals who cancelled or did not appear for their clinic appointment. During the initial home visit and testing of individuals who live alone, the clinical staff also checked the home for potential safety threats, using a standardized checklist that the authors developed. If problems were identified, they were discussed with the individual and, with the individual's approval, the family.

As suggested, the authors incorporated memory screenings into their work in the community. Individuals who were not ready or willing to see a physician for suspected memory problems often felt comfortable having a free check-up. Once the screening and brief medical history were completed, all information on individuals who performed lower than norms for the given tests was reviewed by clinic physician, and a decision was made regarding follow-up neuropsychologic testing. If the physician decided that further testing was warranted, an in-home appointment for the testing was scheduled, along with a meeting with the family member who served as the informant. The Uniform Data Set battery of tests used by federally funded ADCs was completed, and the physician again reviewed results to determine who should be scheduled for a complete neurologic workup.

Many cognitive tests are culturally and educationally biased. Consequently, African Americans and those with low education levels may score low on these tests despite normal cognition, resulting in false-positive results on measures, such as the Mini Mental Status Examination [20]. Recent normative data for older African Americans suggest that the expanded and modified Mini Mental Status Examination (3MSE) is a more sensitive measure with African Americans [21]. The authors have used the 3MSE to screen patients for memory problems since 2005. After review of the literature for measures that might allow the authors to identify early problems with memory in African Americans, they selected the Fuld Object Memory Test [22] as the second screening measure for use in combination with the 3MSE. The authors eliminated other tests from consideration because of a lack of validation with African Americans, strong correlations with education, or excessive time requirements [23–26]. Individuals who scored 77 or lower on the 3MSE and 18 or lower on total retrieval for three administrations of the Fuld Object Memory Test were referred to the clinic physician.

Findings

The accomplishment of AADOP's three objectives required gaining the trust of the African-American community. Without the development of trust, the community would not attend educational presentations and conferences. Without education, older African Americans and their families would not be aware of the early symptoms of dementia and would not request memory check-ups. Without confidence in the quality of available care, persons with memory problems who had received memory check-ups or who were referred by their physicians would not seek clinical evaluations and follow-up care. Further, without trust and confidence, family members would not participate in support groups or use other needed services.

The first evidence that the authors had begun to remove barriers was community participation in their educational activities. When their Branch Out Kentucky conference on AD on a Sunday afternoon in the autumn of 2005 attracted more than 330 participants, most of whom were African American (95%), the authors knew that they had gotten the community's attention related to the health importance of AD. Enthusiasm by the Advisory Council of Ministers for this large conference had grown as they became more informed about the health impact of AD. The 2005 conference focused on the importance of early diagnosis and treatment, innovative counseling techniques with patients and family members, creative caregiver solutions to difficult behaviors, and the importance of African-American participation in research.

Building on information from the conference, caregiver responses, and encouragement and direction from the ministers, a resource document, *The Book of Alzheimer's Disease for African American Churches*, was written so that the program's church partners would have a readily available guide for their church libraries. This resource publication was suggested by the ministers and reviewed by them, and it includes a chapter on the importance of maintaining the patient's spirituality. Surprisingly, the book has been requested by communities across the nation. Brochures explaining clinic services and providing contact information were printed and have been widely distributed in the local community.

The authors have made more than 150 presentations reaching more than 7000 individuals since 2003. These numbers include four local conferences, one designed specifically for ministers and their wives and church health leaders. Administrators and staff at retirement communities and nursing facilities serving African Americans were offered small group lectures on the symptoms of AD, and memory check-ups were offered to group members and their clients. With the increased visibility that presentations, publications, and conferences provided the AADOP, instead of staff making calls to request a time for presentations and memory check-ups, groups were calling the AADOP. African-American graduate students and volunteers were trained on testing techniques that screened for the need for further cognitive testing and neurologic evaluation and assisted with the memory check-ups.

In the authors' work in the community, they found that when discussions of AD and dementia were framed in terms of personal safety, families more readily accepted the message than when the disease symptoms were approached directly. The authors emphasized the warning signs of AD in terms of how these symptoms affected the individual's personal safety and ability to live alone in family meetings and in promotional materials.

With the relationships established through the AADOP, the number of patients being cared for at the clinic increased dramatically over 4 years. The clinic, operating 1 day per week with two physicians, currently serves more than 100 primarily African-American patients (82% of clinic patients) each year. An open house at the clinic has been held yearly to introduce and reinforce the program's community presence. At the 2003 open house event, 45 persons were screened for problems with memory, with more than half requiring follow-up testing. Even though the open house did not begin until 10:00 AM, people were standing in line at 9:30 AM. Many had found out about the event through their churches.

The most frequent diagnosis at the clinic has been AD (52%), with mild cognitive impairment, the earliest detectable form of memory loss, the largest other group of patients evaluated (28%). The mean age of patients was 76.8 years, and, generally, the patient population was less educated than individuals in other programs at the UK's ADC. Approximately 20% have 8 years or less of education, and 64% have 12 years or less.

Sixty-six in-home safety checks were conducted for individuals with suspected memory loss who were living alone. The most common outcome associated with safety checks (21% of cases) was for the family to become aware that were was a medical problem and to increase their involvement with the older person's daily care, often acquiring power of attorney.

A total of 330 individuals received free memory check-ups at various community sites. Of those individuals receiving memory screenings, approximately 180 (53%) required further evaluation through the memory clinic. A surprising finding was that a larger than expected proportion of those screened (15%) were found to have mild cognitive impairment, often an early precursor of AD. The authors' earlier experience in the clinic was that most African-American patients who had AD were identified in the moderate to severe stage of disease. Identifying individuals early by screening and outreach enabled patients to benefit fully from available medications and have meaningful involvement in planning their own future care. This was an important goal of the program.

Offering counseling and support to family members and friends who care for those with dementia was a part of the overall program goal. Before the AADOP was created, African Americans did not attend support groups offered through the local Alzheimer's association. Even after the authors identified an African-American facilitator and formed a new group, only one or two persons attended each month. The authors brought this lack of participation to their advisory groups, and the advisory groups suggested a name change to "Fellowship Hour," because, they explained, "African Americans are very independent and do not want to acknowledge a need for support." The authors changed the name to Fellowship Hour, and membership soared. The evening group has 25 active members, and a second requested daytime group has 3 to 6 members, with participants driving from surrounding counties to attend.

Five lessons learned

1. Keep the program design flexible, and seek community input. The authors used focus groups and advisory councils to guide program development and to evaluate what they were doing. Careful listening and a clear response from the program to what is heard were key elements of this approach. The original outreach strategy was changed several times to fit local culture and needs based on such feedback. For example, the authors had not planned educational conferences with national-caliber speakers for a layperson audience; however, the Advisory Council of Ministers recommended conferences, and, with their sanction, the conferences were extremely successful and allowed the program to reach larger audiences than possible without them. Ongoing evaluation and use of feedback from the served population were critical. This clinical outreach would not have worked had the authors not listened to the community.

2. Keep language simple, and avoid the use of terminology specific to the medical field before the community is educated about dementia. The authors used the advisory councils to review flyers, brochures, and resource materials. One of the initial brochures used "cognitive impairment," terminology that is standard in the authors' work. Council members immediately commented that such jargon was not standard or understandable to the community that the authors were attempting to reach. Cognitive impairment was replaced with "problems with memory and thinking," a simple but critical change. Similar potential language barriers were corrected because of suggestions from the advisory councils.

3. Education can combat the negative stigma associated with dementia and remove the code of silence often practiced by African Americans and their families. Mental health problems in the African-American community are often hidden because families are embarrassed. The community learned that changes in behavior and personality that accompany AD and other forms of dementia are caused by diseases of the brain and require medical attention and treatment.

4. Education can increase the early identification of African Americans with AD and related dementias. Memory screenings by trained staff with measures appropriate to the population can offer reassurance to those who are concerned about changes in memory that their changes are normal and can offer the advantages of early identification to others who have changes significant enough to warrant follow-up treatment and care.

5. When feasible, involve families, not just the primary caregiver, in the care process. In African-American families, decision making often involves multiple individuals from extended family and friendship networks. Respect for older persons is strong and may be shown by

attention to how decisions are made for them. Families should be told that seeking health care support for their older family members is not disrespectful but allows the older person with disease to improve his or her personal safety and have a better quality of life.

References

[1] Gorelick PB, Freels S, Harris Y, et al. Epidemiology of vascular and Alzheimer's dementia among African Americans in Chicago, IL baseline frequency and comparison of risk factors. Neurology 1994;44:1391–6.

[2] Hendrie HC, Ogunniyi A, Hall KS, et al. Incidence of dementia and Alzheimer's disease in two communities: Yoruba residing in Ibadan, Nigeria, and African Americans residing in Indianapolis, Indiana. JAMA 2001;285:739–47.

[3] Heyman A, Fillenbaum G, Prosnitz B, et al. Estimated prevalence of dementia among elderly black and white community residents. Arch Neurol 1991;48:594–8.

[4] Nyenhuis DL, Gorelick PB, Freels S, et al. Cognitive and functional decline in African American with VaD, AD, and stroke without dementia. Neurology 2002;58:56–61.

[5] Fitzpatrick AL, Kuller LH, Ives DG, et al. Incidence and prevalence of dementia in the cardiovascular health study. J Am Geriatr Soc 2004;52:195–204.

[6] Janevic MR, Connell CM. Racial, ethnic and cultural differences in the dementia caregiving experience. Gerontologist 2001;41:334–7.

[7] Connell CM, Shaw BA, Holmes SB, et al. Caregivers' attitudes toward their family members' participation in Alzheimer's disease research: implications for recruitment and retention. Alzheimer Dis Assoc Disord 2001;15:137–45.

[8] Chen M, Fernandex HL. How important are risk factors in Alzheimer's disease? J Alzheimers Dis 2000;2:119–21.

[9] Herbert LE, Scherr PA, Bienias JL, et al. Alzheimer's disease in the US population: prevalence estimates using the 2000 census. Arch Neurol 2003;60:1119–22.

[10] Cooper R, Rotimi C, Ataman S, et al. The prevalence of hypertension in seven populations of West African origin. Am J Public Health 1997;87:160–8.

[11] Bhargava D, Weiner MF, Hynan LS, et al. Vascular disease and risk factors, rate of progression and survival in Alzheimer's disease. J Geriatr Psychiatry Neurol 2007;19(2):78–82.

[12] Green RC, Cupples LA, Go R, et al. Risk of dementia among white and African American relatives of patients with Alzheimer's disease. JAMA 2002;237(3):329–36.

[13] Froehlich TE, Bogardus ST, Inouye SK. Dementia and race: are there differences between African Americans and Caucasians? J Am Geriatr Soc 2001;49:477–84.

[14] Ogunniyi A, Hall KS, Gureje O, et al. Risk factors for incident Alzheimer's disease in African Americans and Yoruba. Metab Brain Dis 2006;21(2–3):224–9.

[15] Levkoff S, Levy B, Weitzman PF. The role of religion and ethnicity in the help seeking of family caregivers of elders with Alzheimer's disease and related disorders. J Cross Cult Gerontol 1999;14:335–56.

[16] Cox C. Race and caregiving: patterns of service use by African American and white caregivers of persons with Alzheimer's disease. J Gerontol Soc Work 1999;32(2):5–19.

[17] Dilworth-Anderson P, Gibson B. Cultural influence of values, norms, meanings and perceptions in understanding dementia in ethnic minorities. Alzheimer Dis Assoc Disord 2003;16: S56–63.

[18] Shavers VL, Lynch CF, Burmeister LF. Knowledge of the Tuskegee study and its impact on willingness to participate in medical research studies. J Natl Med Assoc 2000;92:563–72.

[19] Jones JH. Bad blood: the Tuskegee syphilis experiment. 2nd edition. New York: Free Press; 1993.

[20] Folstein MF, Folstein SE, McHugh PR. Mini Mental State: a practical method for grading state of patients for the clinician. J Psychiatr Res 1975;12:189–98.

[21] Brown LM, Schinka JA, Mortimer JA, et al. 3MS normative data for elderly African Americans. J Clin Exp Neuropsychol 2003;25:234–41.

[22] Fuld PA. Guaranteed stimulus processing in the evaluation of memory and learning. Cortex 1980;16:255–71.

[23] Whitfield KE. Challenges in cognitive assessment of African Americans in research on Alzheimer's disease. Alzheimer Dis Assoc Disord 2002;16(Suppl 2):S80–1.

[24] Mast BT, Fitzgerald J, Steinberg J, et al. Effective screening for Alzheimer's disease among older African Americans. Clin Neuropsychol 2001;15:196–202.

[25] Green RC, Clarke VC, Thompson NJ, et al. Early detection of Alzheimer's disease: methods, markers, and misgiving. Alzheimer Dis Assoc Disord 1997;11(Suppl 5):S1–5 [discussion: S37–9].

[26] Ford GR, Haley WE, Thrower SL. Utility of Mini Mental State exam scores in predicting functional impairment among white and African American dementia patients. J Gerontol A Biol Sci Med Sci 1996;51:M185–8.

ELSEVIER
SAUNDERS

Nurs Clin N Am 43 (2008) 449–467

NURSING
CLINICS
OF NORTH AMERICA

Maternal and Newborn Care During Disasters: Thinking Outside the Hospital Paradigm

Jeanne Pfeiffer, RN, MPH, CIC[a],*,
Melissa D. Avery, PhD, CNM, FACNM[a],
Mary Benbenek, MS, RN, FNP, PNP[a],
Robbie Prepas, CNM, MN, JD[b],
Lisa Summers, CNM, MSN, DrPH[c],
Cecilia M. Wachdorf, PhD, CNM[a],
Carol O'Boyle, PhD, RN[a]

[a]*School of Nursing, University of Minnesota, 308 Harvard Street SE,
Minneapolis, MN 55455, USA*
[b]*Nurse Practitioner Program, UCLA-Harbor Medical Center,
740 Oak Street, Laguna Beach, CA 92651, USA*
[c]*American College of Nurse Midwives, 1220 Noyes Drive,
Silver Spring, MD 20910, USA*

During and immediately following public health disasters, primary emphasis is placed on meeting the immediate needs of disaster victims. These include food, shelter, decontamination, trauma care, antibiotics, or respiratory support, depending on the type of disaster. Routine health care needs of vulnerable populations may not be recognized or specifically addressed in planning. Pregnant women, new mothers, and their infants constitute such vulnerable populations that warrant predisaster planning.

In 2005 following Hurricane Katrina, The Washington Post reported that 125 critically ill newborn babies and 154 pregnant women were evacuated to Woman's Hospital in Baton Rouge without their medical records [1].

This project was supported under the Minnesota Emergency Readiness Education and Training Program funded by a grant from the Assistant Secretary of Preparedness and Response under Health and Human Services.

* Corresponding author.

E-mail address: pfeif052@umn.edu (J. Pfeiffer).

Robbie Prepas, CNM, member of a Disaster Medical Assistance Team that participated in Hurricane Katrina, attended several births in the New Orleans airport [1]. In Minneapolis, Minnesota on August 1, 2007, one of the first victims evacuated from the interstate 35W bridge collapse was a pregnant woman who had sustained internal injuries and required an emergency caesarean section [2]. On October 22, 2007 San Bernardino County (SBC), California initiated an evacuation in response to fires in the Grass Valley and Slide areas, forcing people to leave their homes. In the week following the fires, pregnant women (SBC officials did not have exact numbers), either in active labor or who needed medical evaluation, were among the 1000 individuals who were evacuated and treated in a temporary clinic space assigned to the Medical Reserve Corps within the Red Cross evacuee shelter at the National Orange Show Festival Grounds [3].

Historically during disasters, whether natural or manmade, there is a tendency to focus on the needs of the general population and not specifically on the needs of special populations, such as pregnant, birthing, postpartum, and lactating women and their newborns. Because pregnancy, birth, and early postpartum are perceived to be normal physiologic events, it may be assumed that no preparations are needed. Provision of prenatal care and accurate triage to safe places for birth and newborn care are critical to minimizing morbidity and mortality for these two groups. Providing safe care to these populations in low-resource temporary care environments, such as churches, schools, tents, trailers, and convention centers, following disasters requires a great deal of planning and creativity.

This article explores the needs of pregnant, laboring, and postpartum women and newborn infants during disasters within the context of care normally delivered to these populations. Many communities have general disaster plans; however, few have specific plans for the care of these intimately linked special populations during prolonged events [4]. Stimulation of ideas, discussion, and creative problem solving helps address the planning, education of disaster response teams, and provision of appropriate supplies and equipment needed for these special populations.

It is estimated that roughly 56,000 women and 75,000 infants were affected by Hurricane Katrina [5]. The magnitude of that disaster serves to demonstrate the potentially large number of women and children who might be affected by public health disasters in which there is a loss of public infrastructures and limited access to health care and other life necessities, such as water, food, medications, and shelter. Table 1 provides recent data on the number of births per day in the United States and the state of Minnesota, including the number of caesarean sections, infants born prematurely, infants of low birth weight, and the number of maternal and newborn deaths.

Appropriate "what if" questions that might be asked when developing plans for the care of pregnant women and newborns during a public health disaster, such as the SBC fires, include: How will women in labor be triaged?

Table 1
2006 United States and Minnesota natality statistics

Categories	United states no. (%)	Minnesota no. (%)
Births	4,265,996 (NC) = 11,687/d [6]	73,515 (NC) = 201/d [7]
Caesarean births	1,326,725 (31.1%) = 3,635/d [6]	18,673 (25.4%) = 51/d [7]
Low birth weight babies (<2500 g)	354,078 (8.3%) = 970/d [6]	4,852 (6.6%) = 13/d [7]
Premature	546,047 (12.8%) = 1496/d [6]	7,719 (10.5%) = 21/d [7]
Neonatal deaths	18,275[a] (NC) = 50/d [8]	243 (NC) = 5/wk [9]
Maternal deaths	12.1/100,000 live births[b] (NC) [10]	5 (NC) [11]

Abbreviation: NC, not computed.
[a] 2003 figure.
[b] 2001 figure.

Where will they give birth? Are birth kits available? Can the newborns be cared for at this location? Are the shelter facilities adequate for all births? What additional interventions should have been planned to care for these women and their newborns? How will pregnant women in early or midterm pregnancy receive the ongoing care they need? Is the number of pregnant women residing in the area known? How many can be expected to give birth before the disaster is under control? How many newborns (birth to 28 days) are in the area and will need support? The following discussion begins to answer these questions and set the stage for ongoing planning and education to care for pregnant women and infants in times of public health emergencies.

Transfer of operations to national incident command during a disaster

Valuable lessons have been learned from recent natural disasters and from acts of terrorism. Most emergencies are best handled locally, but when major events, such as floods, hurricanes, intentional destruction of people and property, or pandemics occur, it is necessary to seek help from other jurisdictions through mutual aid agreements. The National Integration Center was established in 2003 under order of President Bush per Section 502 of the Homeland Security Act 6 U.S.C. §§ 101 et seq., Homeland Security Presidential Directive 5 by the Secretary of Homeland Security to provide strategic direction for and oversight of the National Incident Management System (NIMS). The NIMS is a system that provides order when responding to catastrophic events using a command and control infrastructure that is set up immediately within all affected government and community agencies (including hospitals) responding to the event. This elaborate command system expands and contracts in response to the magnitude of the public health emergency. The NIMS may trigger many functions within one agency or multiple agencies within the affected location. Agencies are expected to work within a unified command agreement to manage the disaster [12]. Nurses and other health care providers in the United States are being educated and trained in use of criteria for activating and functioning within the hospital incident command system (HICS). Decisions are made about the personnel job descriptions best qualified by knowledge and skills within a health care system to fill a specific HICS function in the command center or in one of the supporting (eg, finance, logistics, operations, or planning) divisions. In addition, systems are being instituted and tested to alert all staff by fax, email, cell phone, or home phone to respond to an emergency at the hospital. Through the Area Command Center, hospitals are participating in multiagency exercises to improve coordination with other community agencies. As an example, this coordinated effort allows communities to obtain assistance from other jurisdictions to provide adequate staffing. Essentially this coordinated, standardized approach provides access to resources when disaster has depleted those resources within a community [13].

During a prolonged event, it is expected that caring for a large number of patients will occur in non–hospital-based settings. Pregnant, birthing, and postpartum mothers with their newborns are two intimately linked special populations that would benefit greatly from expertise of care providers who plan before a hazardous event occurs.

Planners and providers from acute care, public health, emergency management, and emergency medical services should craft and rehearse the "preferred plan." Rehearsal with all collaborators would facilitate provision of care in improvised settings, using the safest possible alternatives during an event [14].

Continuity of care for pregnant women during a disaster

Under normal circumstances, about 99% of births in the United States occur in a hospital or clinical setting [15]. During a public health emergency, it might not be possible or desirable to get to a hospital or clinic [6]. Caring for pregnant women during prolonged events, such as pandemic influenza or a terrorist event, represents a unique situation when women may not have access to a hospital or to their primary care provider [4]. Knowledge about routine care during pregnancy, labor, birth, and the postpartum period helps responders to understand and anticipate the potential impact of the unmet needs of pregnant women. Although pregnancy is generally considered a normal physiologic and developmental event, the increased stress women can experience during a disaster situation may result in preterm labor, low birth weight, and other high-risk situations, as seen after September 11, 2001 (World Trade Center attack) in New York, after August 29, 2005 in Louisiana (Hurricane Katrina), and following the tsunami in Indonesia in 2004 [16,17].

Care during the prenatal period begins with an initial visit composed of a complete history, physical examination, routine laboratory tests, and careful dating of the pregnancy. Health history components include family medical history, including genetic information, and a complete past medical history of the pregnant woman. Menstrual history is important in dating the pregnancy, and for women who have been pregnant previously, past obstetric history is included. Any risk factors are noted and a physical examination follows. Uterine sizing, combined with menstrual data, provides the first information about current pregnancy dating and an estimation of the due date [18].

Laboratory tests, such as blood type and Rh factor, hemoglobin, urinalysis, and appropriate genetic and infectious disease tests (eg, cystic fibrosis and hepatitis), occur at the first visit. At approximately 24 to 28 weeks' gestation, women are screened for anemia and gestational diabetes; antibody testing for Rh-negative women is performed so they can receive RhoGAM as needed [18,19]. Immunizations, such as influenza (inactive), hepatitis B, and tetanus, may also be recommended during pregnancy depending on the individual situation [20]. Providing the complete pregnancy database to women as a personal health record is ideal because when a disaster occurs, access to the regular medical records may not be possible.

Ongoing maternal and fetal health status is monitored throughout pregnancy by evaluation of laboratory studies, maternal blood pressure, weight gain, and fundal height measurements, and by observing the fetal heart rate, discussing fetal activity levels, and determining cervical changes and fetal position as appropriate. These measurements and observations typically provide reassurance to the practitioner and mother that the pregnancy is progressing normally but are also used to determine if a problem exists. Special guidance and counseling are provided to women who had a previous Caesarean section. In addition, RhoGAM must be available to women during pregnancy and postbirth as appropriate to prevent future isoimmunization [21].

When a disaster occurs, providers must triage pregnant women according to risk status. Women must be identified according to those who have essentially normal pregnancies requiring basic care and ongoing support, those who might need a higher level of surveillance, and women who have high-risk pregnancies requiring specialized care. The most common abnormal conditions diagnosed during pregnancy are hypertension, preterm labor, and gestational diabetes [19]. Providers should be aware of increased risk for complications, such as preterm labor and intrauterine growth retardation [22]. Infections can be more severe in pregnant women because of the physiologic immunosuppression that occurs in pregnancy [23].

During events caused by an infectious disease agent, medications normally used to treat infections or immunizations to prevent infections, such as live attenuated vaccines, may not be safely administered to pregnant women because of the potential for harm to the fetus [20]. Finally, some researchers have examined the effects from toxins, stress, and radiation and found adverse effects on the unborn child [23].

Although the frequency of contact with a provider may be altered during an emergency, the essential needs of pregnant women that must be met include: adequate food, water, and rest in a safe, clean environment; access to ongoing prenatal care and knowledgeable health care providers who can direct care when complications occur; and access to social and mental health services. Pregnant women and their families may need information about which of the limited food products available during a crisis may be most important for their nutrition. In addition to nutrition and weight gain, guidance is provided to women on topics related to normal changes to expect during pregnancy, family involvement in care, preparation for labor and birth, and plans for care of the newborn and support for the new mother at home [22,24]. Counseling regarding caloric intake, specific nutrient components of food intake, prenatal vitamins, and any other supplements, such as calcium, hydration, weight gain, and physical activity, are ongoing components of comprehensive prenatal care, essential to a woman's own health and the growth and development of her fetus.

Care during labor and birth is primarily supportive and includes providing assessment and assurance of normal progress, monitoring maternal vital signs and fetal heart rate, providing nutrition and hydration as appropriate, and providing physical and emotional support to promote comfort as labor progresses. Pharmacologic support may be required depending on maternal status and labor progress and her particular preferences for care. Additional interventions may be required based on individual needs and maternal and fetal condition.

When a disaster occurs, triage related to place of birth is superimposed on the customary assessment processes that occur under ordinary circumstances. Plans should be in place to have simple birth packs containing required equipment to support normal birth, using less technology than is available in hospital settings. At home or in other low-resource settings, common pharmacologic support methods promoting comfort in labor are unlikely to be available; therefore, care providers and supportive others must be prepared to use additional means of supporting women in labor, such as back rubs, slow rhythmic breathing, light abdominal massage (effleurage), position changes, and encouraging human presence [25]. Spouses or significant others and family members should be prepared to support the needs of the woman in labor and giving birth with limited presence of health care workers [19,25].

Support of normal processes and assessment for deviations continues in the postpartum period. Monitoring vital signs, bleeding, and signs of infection, and maintenance of adequate nutrition, hydration, and comfort are important considerations. Emotional status is evaluated along with normal physiologic changes following birth. Women are assisted to feed and care for their infants. When breastfeeding is the method of choice, additional education regarding nutrition, hydration, rest, physical activity, and feeding techniques is necessary. A discussion about family planning method and desired child spacing is typically initiated during pregnancy and discussed again with resources and any pharmacologic methods or devices provided in the postpartum period.

Postpartum care and support of lactation are other critical areas to plan for in disaster situations. The Centers for Disease Control and Prevention recommends the continuation of breastfeeding after a natural disaster and the re-establishment of exclusive breastfeeding to prevent infections associated with sanitation and interruption of the supply of clean water for drinking and bathing [26]. Mothers who are not breastfeeding need assistance to place the infant at the breast. Those combining breast and formula feeding can more easily return to exclusive breastfeeding.

Because postpartum depression, psychosis, and posttraumatic stress disorder are more common during disaster situations, availability of mental health providers is essential to help with assessment of women's mental health status and support stress reduction [27].

Additional special circumstances for women include the health care needs of those who wish to avoid an unintended pregnancy, which can be associated with increased maternal morbidity [28]. Maintaining physical safety is critical [29] to prevent and manage the consequences of sexual and gender-based violence that can occur following a disaster [5]. According to the World Health Organization in the Health Action in Crises Forum (2006) "Crisis situations and emergencies place pregnant women and newborns at even greater risk for adverse outcomes because of the sudden and prolonged loss of medical support, increased cases of trauma, malnutrition, disease, and exposure to violence" [30]. Providing adequate shelter against the elements and protecting from violence are essential tasks during disaster conditions.

Continuity of care for newborns

Newborn health is closely linked to maternal health. Newborn care providers must be aware of the maternal health and prenatal history, including any risk factors, such as multifetal gestation, infection, preterm labor, a fetus that is small or large for gestational age, and any other maternal medical conditions. Maintenance of a clean environment and taking precautions against infection are basic care elements.

Typically 80% of newborns are classified as healthy. Characteristics of a healthy newborn include: normal pregnancy and delivery; full-term birth (greater than 37 weeks' gestation); appearance (color), pulse, grimace, activity, and respiratory (APGAR) scores of seven or more at 5 minutes of life and no resuscitation needed; birth weight between the 10th and 90th percentiles; no signs of soft tissue wasting; no obvious congenital abnormalities or physical findings; and feeding and breathing with no apparent problems [31,32]. In a disaster situation, these same criteria can and should be used as a quick measure of newborn health.

Full head-to-toe physical examination is necessary at birth. Ongoing assessment to identify clinical findings consistent with wellness in the neonatal period (first 28 days of life) is also important. Normal clinical findings include pink skin, body temperature greater than 37°C, 30 to 60 respirations/min, occasional cry, good suckling with establishment of breast feeding, passing of stool and urine within 24 hours, and heart rate of 100 to 160 beats/min [33,34]. Most newborns lose up to 10% of their weight in the first few days after birth and should regain this weight by 2 weeks postpartum. Even in low-resource settings, caregivers can perform this examination and continue to monitor the stability of the newborn.

Essentials of newborn care under normal circumstances include: safe environment; promotion of maternal–infant bonding; establishment and maintenance of airway, breathing, and circulation; facilitation of thermoregulation; establishment and maintenance of breastfeeding; prevention and detection of infections; prevention of neonatal bleeding; administration of immunizations; and special attention to low birth weight and sick infants [18,33,35–37]. Providing a safe environment with trained personnel and the equipment necessary to intervene in the event of complications is typically the role of the hospital, including resuscitation of the infant if needed and assurance that airway, breathing, and circulation are maintained. In a disaster setting, the essentials of newborn care must be maintained, even if the birth site and environment might change drastically.

Newborns must receive care as early as possible to implement preventive interventions, such as eye infection prophylaxis, vaccination, and vitamin K. Early identification of abnormalities facilitates referrals of at-risk newborns to tertiary care settings. Conditions requiring referral include: extremely low birth weight (<1500 g), respiratory distress, seizures or unconscious infant, hypothermia, severe pallor, jaundice within the first 24 hours, severe birth injury, severe congenital abnormalities, inability to pass urine or stool within 24 hours, somnolent or very irritable infant, and inability to feed [31].

Early establishment of breastfeeding in newborns is strongly recommended [36,38–41] and should begin within the first hour of birth, ideally continuing beyond 6 months [41]. In fact, exclusive breastfeeding in normal circumstances can have a positive influence on infant health in a disaster as compared with infants who are given free breast milk substitutes when they are not indicated [42]. Breast milk does not require a water source to prepare, so offers protection from diarrheal illnesses, which can occur during disaster because of water contamination.

The promotion of maternal–infant bonding is a primary goal during disaster. Facilitating immediate skin-to-skin contact using kangaroo mother care and infant massage can be useful [36,43]. Kangaroo mother care is a technique originally developed to promote thermoregulation in premature infants. The baby is placed against the mother's skin, between the breasts, and then mother and infant are covered, holding the infant in place. This useful, easily implemented technique can be used in place of an incubator during a disaster.

The most common causes of newborn death include infection; congenital malformations; prematurity-related disorders; complications of membranes, placenta, or umbilical cord; respiratory distress; neonatal hemorrhage; and diseases of the circulatory system [44,45]. Careful ongoing observation of changes in skin color, temperature, signs of infection, feeding, and elimination is necessary to identify early evidence of these conditions. Basic thermoregulation can be supported by use of the "warm chain" as described in Women and Infants Service Project (WISP), including essential items such as clothing and blankets and other supportive processes (Box 1).

It is critical following birth during a disaster to assure that the infant is clearly and accurately identified and placed with the mother. If the infant requires transport to a hospital or transfer to a regional treatment center, it is imperative that the place of transport be accurately and clearly communicated to mother and family. The response to Hurricane Katrina revealed flaws in current systems of transfer and identified the need for a system of communication that allows for prompt notification of site of transfer to parents and accurate report of clinical condition to the receiving center [47,48].

Recommendations

Advance planning to meet maternal and newborn needs during a disaster

Although women and infants are disproportionately affected by emergencies, local, state, and national programs have not adequately addressed the needs of these two populations [4] in their hazard vulnerability analysis for a given locale [5]. Consideration of the population in a specific jurisdiction

---

Box 1. The warm chain [46]

Warm delivery room
Immediate drying
Skin-to-skin contact
Breastfeeding
Bathing and weighing postponed
Appropriate clothing and bedding
Mother and baby together
Warm transportation
Warm resuscitation
Training/awareness raising

Data from World Health Organization DoRHaRR. Thermal protection of the newborn: a practical guide (WHO/RHT/MSM/97.2). World Health Organization. Available at: http://www.who.int/reproductive-health/publications/MSM_97_2_Thermal_protection_of_the_newborn/. Accessed September 28, 2005.

458   PFEIFFER et al

or geographic area, including awareness of the local or regional birth rate and number of newborns likely to need support in a given period of time, supports planning with evidence of need [49].

Previous disasters have amplified awareness of the need to plan ahead to meet health care needs of pregnant women and newborn infants [4,5,47,50–53]. A National Working Group on Women and Infant Needs in Emergencies (WISP) was created through the White Ribbon Alliance to address the safe delivery of infants worldwide [51]. Internationally, much has been written about improving birth outcomes in the field during disasters. The Indian Academy of Pediatrics [31] drafted disaster management guidelines aimed at minimizing morbidity and mortality for mothers and infants during the perinatal period. Similarly, Save the Children [54] and the March of Dimes [4] developed guidelines to assure maternal and newborn health during disasters and prepared checklists itemizing necessary equipment and supplies. Even earlier the *Journal of Midwifery and Women's Health* published a series of papers regarding the care of women and newborns in low-resource settings. Topics included disaster preparedness, pregnancy and childbirth care in low-resource settings, and newborn care in adverse conditions [14].

A resource for giving birth "in place" [18] specified the use of household items required to assist at birth. The Indian Academy of Pediatrics describes a delivery kit for use by trained field personnel, which includes household items and basic resuscitation equipment [31]. Protocols regarding medications, such as antibiotics, vitamin K, conjunctivitis prevention, and oral rehydration solution, are also recommended for health care workers to use in the field.

Planning for women and infants during disasters must include continuous access to prenatal care, ability to access current health information (such as blood type, immunization status, and any important complications being treated), and appropriate facilities to support labor, birth, and immediate care of postpartum mothers and newborns. Assuring that pregnant women have enough food and hydration supports two lives. Basic sanitation, including disposal of materials containing blood and body fluids, must also be considered. Pregnant women and new mothers and their newborns are typically healthy individuals; protecting and supporting optimal health and avoiding unnecessary exposures to other individuals who have contagious health conditions is paramount.

In some disasters, such as a pandemic influenza outbreak, authors agree that hospitalization will be necessary for some women [55]. Although women may initially think they need to continue to come to the hospital, hospitals will not be the optimal place to care for many healthy women and newborns because of the risk for transmission of disease to these populations [55]. During a pandemic, it is likely that one of the public health strategies to minimize transmission will be social distancing, or minimizing contact between people by canceling public events and closing schools and offices [56]. As part of social distancing, home birth may become preferred for some normal births; therefore, consulting those who have expertise in supporting birth in out-of-hospital settings and preparing hospital-based health care practitioners in advance is an important step. In addition to homes, environments such as churches, schools, tents, equipped portable trailers, convention centers, existing freestanding birth centers, and surgical centers can provide alternatives for care to low-risk women for labor and birth.

Stocking birth and newborn kits based on the average number of births in a region is a step few emergency preparedness teams have considered. Rapid response medical planning teams should include physicians, midwives, and nurses experienced in care of pregnant and postpartum women and newborns from both civilian and military community sources [57].

Triage systems are fundamental in distinguishing between women who need basic supportive care and those who need more complex care. In a situation in which hospitals are not accessible or available or are considered unsafe for healthy pregnant women, health care provider teams need to assess women and newborns to provide the safest level of care in the safest location. Which women can be attended at home by family members? Who can be supported by phone, community resources, or health care providers as available? Who would be best served in a low-risk facility with a higher level of available resources, and who must be transported for hospital care? When hospitalization is necessary, contact between otherwise healthy women and newborns and other contagious individuals must be avoided [58].

Care delivered in an emergency situation requires basic documentation. Births are part of our national vital records system and documentation must be continued during an emergency. Design of a simple personal health record that pregnant women and their families can carry with them will facilitate ongoing care and appropriate triage. State-mandated newborn screening systems must also be continued as much as possible and appropriately documented [53]. When separation of family members is necessary, basic records containing names of patient and immediate family members, contact information for each, and site of transport (receiving facility) are critical documentation elements.

Because of the probability of needing additional care providers during emergencies, "A number of recent laws and agreements have made it easier for medical personnel from other regions to provide health care assistance to affected areas. The need to make the best use of volunteer health workers in an emergency led to the development of the Emergency System for Advance Registration of Health Professions Volunteers (ESARHPV). Each state is currently developing a system to contain up-to-date information about: a volunteer's identity, licensing, credentialing, accreditation and privileging in hospitals or other medical organizations" [59]. The goal is to have a ready group of volunteers who are approved to respond to a request for mutual aid to a specific facility or agency [59].

Education and training for immediate readiness

With an awareness of the needs of pregnant women and newborns, development of education programs should include guidelines suited to the specific setting and a calendar of scheduled exercises to teach the plan and to test the readiness of those who are expected to provide care (eg, workshops, tabletops, drills, simulations /functional and full-scale community exercises) [18]. Components of an effective guideline include triage and care of patients, methods to track and monitor care during the event, and assessment of patients and providers regarding the psychologic impact of the event.

The development of a uniform educational program directed by evidence-based recommendations in a guideline serves several purposes. All stakeholders, including typical health care providers and emergency planners, come to the same forum to develop a framework focusing discussion on these unique populations. The guideline-development process can help identify gaps in resources, systems, knowledge, skills, and ability to establish and operate under the NIMS chain-of-command infrastructure that is expected to be in place during a disaster of any kind [13]. A completed guideline is also an effective communication tool for all stakeholders.

It can be difficult to develop a guideline that fits all hazards, however; hurricanes, ice storms, and floods create different challenges than pandemic influenza. Each state thus needs to conduct a hazard vulnerability analysis, prioritize the most likely hazards, and plan accordingly [60]. All states should include an influenza pandemic in their priorities. National guidelines and local plans should be reviewed and revised at regular intervals for changes that significantly affect practice.

Recognized associations or agencies should lead guideline development and assist with implementation by local experts familiar with the specific needs of the population and the resources of the health care community. For example, hospital-based nurses accustomed to providing care in an urban, tertiary setting have different training needs than emergency medical technicians in a rural setting serving a small community hospital.

Exercises that test the written plans and point to education and training needs are part of a cycle of preparedness. Training exercises include educational seminars, workshops with discussion and scenario-based tabletop training and operations-level drills, functional and full-scale exercises incorporating mock victims, computer simulations, and various other technologies. Homeland Security is currently working with all United States agencies to adopt a standardized approach to planning and evaluating these exercises as a requirement to receive ongoing federal grants [61].

The HICS under NIMS is a vital part of the education and training needed by all health care delivery staff. A strong and supportive command staff is critical to monitor care during an event. The staff assigned to perform duties under the HICS may be working with providers in homes and coordinating care with other providers assigned to skilled care facilities.

There should be an identified medical or obstetric unit leader making clear assignments as to where workers will go and what specific job actions or tasks will be required [62].

In the case of all-hazards preparedness within the HICS and NIMS infrastructure, pretraining assessment should go beyond mere knowledge and care of patients. Family emergency preparedness and psychologic first aid for staff and victims during an event should be included. It is critical to assess the comfort level of staff and patients who are involved in a disaster response. If responders know their own families are being cared for, they are more able to focus on their work. Physical demands placed on providers may be significant and have an impact on their coping abilities. Ensuring that staff has adequate food, water, rest, equipment, and support helps stabilize the team until relief staff can step in [63].

People trained in psychologic first aid (PFA) should be assigned to monitor and support victims and people responding to a disaster. "PFA was developed to assist people in the immediate aftermath of disaster and terrorism to reduce initial distress, and to foster short and long-term adaptive functioning. It has been developed for use by mental health specialists including first responders, incident command systems, primary and emergency health care providers, school crisis response teams, faith-based organizations, disaster relief organizations, Community Emergency Response Teams, Medical Reserve Corps, and the Citizens Corps in diverse settings" [64].

Emergency care providers on the scene

Pregnant women, newborns, and infants have unique health care needs during and after a disaster [4]. The goal for educators and trainers involved with pregnant women and newborns is to prepare staff to work with less technology in a low-resource setting. Many health care providers have the challenge of transferring their skills out of the hospital setting and providing a safe environment for out-of-hospital birth [18]. Specific examples of low-tech assessment are palpation of contractions by hand, listening to the fetal heart with a stethoscope, and observing the mother's demeanor for signs of labor progress. Health care providers must be able to accurately evaluate pregnancy-related conditions and appropriately triage pregnant women for immediate care to a safe shelter or health care facility, referring high-risk patients who have complications to acute care facilities [5]. Improvisation is a necessary skill for emergency personnel because there will likely be substantial disruption in the public health and clinical care hierarchy.

In an emergency setting in which technology is limited, it is vital to have the ability to monitor the maternal and fetal condition and assess and treat obstetric conditions. Women and newborns must be screened for complications and referrals initiated for those requiring specialized care. A mechanism for managing complications is essential if birth is imminent or there is an inability to transfer the mother or baby. In addition all health care

Box 2. Birth bag supplies

Sterile tray with instruments, gloves, sterile plastic umbilical
    clamps
Doppler, fetoscope, blood pressure cuff, stethoscope
Resuscitation equipment (O_2, suction, Ambu bag)
Suturing supplies
Intravenous supplies
Scale, blood collection tubes, catheters
Satellite phone
Job aid—laminated card
Infant hat
Lubrication jelly
Plastic bag for placenta
Receiving blanket and disposable towels
Warm clothes for infant appropriate to environment

Data from March of Dimes. Women and infants service package: national
working group for women and infant needs in emergencies in the United States.
The White Ribbon Alliance web site 2007. Available at: http://www.whiteribbonal-
liance.org/Resources/Documents/WISP.Final.07.27.07.pdf. Accessed January 15,
2008.

Box 3. Parent supplies

Sources of heat, light, water
Food and fluids
Bed pads, gauze pads, bulb syringes
Emergency plans and medical records
Clear firm surfaces and cleaning supplies
A thermometer
One newborn hat
One bulb syringe
Six packs of sterile lubricant
Warm clothes for infant appropriate to environment

Data from March of Dimes. Women and infants service package: national
working group for women and infant needs in emergencies in the United States.
The White Ribbon Alliance web site 2007. Available at: http://www.whiteribbonal-
liance.org/Resources/Documents/WISP.Final.07.27.07.pdf. Accessed January 15,
2008; with permission.

providers or emergency professionals should have a working knowledge of neonatal resuscitation [65].

There needs to be an acute awareness of the different roles of the responders; this is always a challenge in a disaster environment in which the situations are often disorganized or chaotic. Professionals may be asked to participate in care outside of their area of expertise; preplanning establishes credentialing for rapid response teams that include people who have the appropriate skill sets to direct care in low-resource settings for this population [5,66]. Many states have formulated legislation for immediate credentialing of out-of-state providers [59].

Non-obstetric health care providers, medical assistant teams, and emergency medical services personnel may need to be prepared to triage pregnant women and make decisions about their care [5]. Women who require advanced-level care in hospitals include those who need caesarean sections or blood transfusions and those who have preterm labor or pregnancy-induced hypertension or diabetes [4]. All care givers should be equipped with basic personal protective equipment to minimize their own exposure to blood and body fluids [14]. Providers and families need readily available birthing and newborn supplies distributed in clinics and in the community. Suggested items are included in Boxes 2 and 3.

Disasters involving pregnant women and newborns have not been addressed adequately in most states since Hurricane Katrina. Planning ahead mitigates maternal and newborn complications and facilitates the provision of effective treatment and use of resources for rapid disaster response. Health care providers, including midwives, physicians, and nurses, can be important resources to meet the needs of this vulnerable population [14].

Summary

Pregnant and laboring women and their newborns constitute vulnerable populations during a disaster. Recognizing and implementing the essentials of pregnancy, postpartum, and newborn care under less-than-desirable circumstances is an ongoing, but not insurmountable, challenge. NIMS provides the standardized organizational framework to create and mobilize rapid-response teams with the skill and expertise necessary to address the needs of these populations. Emphasizing the theme of "clean, warm, and safe" in addition to appropriate triage is integral to planning. Local, state, and national agencies must prioritize the care of women and their infants during a disaster in their policy and procedure development to assure appropriate preparedness for the future.

Acknowledgment

We acknowledge research assistants Bufford Ang and Nivedita Girotra for the formatting of the manuscript.

References

[1] Lakshmi R. Group urges disaster planning for pregnant women, babies. The Washington Post August 17, 2006; Page A09. Available at: http://www.washingtonpost.com/wp-dyn/content/article/2006/08/16/AR2006081601516.html. Accessed January 15, 2008.

[2] Baram M. A glimmer of hope amid the devastation 2007. Available at: http://www.abcnews.go.com/Technology/Story?id=3450574&page=1. Accessed January 14, 2008.

[3] Fire crisis—October 2007: San Bernardino County Medical Reserve Corps renders care to over 1000 at evacuee shelter. SBC MRC Press Release 2007. Available at: www.sbcms.org/mrc. Accessed January 14, 2008.

[4] March of Dimes. Women and infants service package: national working group for women and infant needs in emergencies in the United States. The White Ribbon Alliance web site. 2007. Available at: http://www.whiteribbonalliance.org/Resources/Documents/WISP.Final.07.27.07.pdf. Accessed January 15, 2008.

[5] Callaghan WM, Rasmussen SA, Jamieson DJ, et al. Health concerns of women and infants in times of natural disasters: lessons learned from Hurricane Katrina. Matern Child Health J 2007;11:307–11.

[6] Centers for Disease Control and Prevention. Division of reproductive health: activities —maternal health, infant health, and preterm delivery. 2006. Available at: http://www.cdc.gov/reproductivehealth/DRH/activities/MHIHPD.html. Accessed December 30, 2007.

[7] MN Dept of Health. 2006 Minnesota Health Statistics Annual Summary. Selected live births: Table 2. 2007. Available at: http://www.health.state.mn.us/divs/chs/06annsum/Natality06.pdf. Accessed December 30, 2007.

[8] Centers for Disease Control and Prevention. Infant, neonatal and postneonatal deaths and mortality rates: mother's Hispanic origin and race of mother for non-Hispanic origin by age of mother: United States, 2001 period data. (N.D.) table 61. Available at: http://www.cdc.gov/nchs/data/dvs/LINK01WK61.pdf. Accessed December 30, 2007.

[9] MN Dept of Health. 2006 Minnesota Health Statistics Annual Summary. 2007. Infant mortality and fetal deaths: Table 3. Available at: http://www.health.state.mn.us/divs/chs/06annsum/InfantFetal06.pdf. Accessed December 30, 2007.

[10] Hoyert DL. Maternal mortality and related concepts. National Center for Health Statistics. Vital Health Stat 2007;3(33):1–13. Available at: http://www.cdc.gov/nchs/data/series/sr_03/sr03_033.pdf. Accessed December 30, 2007.

[11] MN Dept of Health. 2006 Minnesota Health Statistics Annual Summary. 2007. Mortality: Table 1. Available at: http://www.health.state.mn.us/divs/chs/06annsum/Mortality06.pdf. Accessed December 30, 2007.

[12] Department of homeland security management directive system: National Incident Management System Integration Center. NIMS Online.com. 2004. Available at: http://www.nimsonline.com/integration_center_directive.htm. Accessed January 14, 2008.

[13] Department of Homeland Security Management Directive System: FEMA: National Incident Management Systems. 2007. Available at: http://www.fema.gov/emergency/nims/. Accessed January 14, 2008.

[14] Keeney GB. Resources for providing care for women and infants in disasters and low-resource settings. J Midwifery Womens Health 2004;49:42–5.

[15] Curtin SC, Park MM. Trends in the attendant, place, and timing of births, and in the use of obstetric interventions: United States, 1989–97. Natl Vital Stat Rep 1999;47:1–12.

[16] Berkowitz GS, Wolff MS, Janevic TM, et al. The effects of the World Trade Center Disaster and intrauterine growth restriction. JAMA 2003;290(5):595–6.

[17] Carballo M, Hernandez M, Schneider K, et al. Impact of the tsunami on reproductive health. International Center for Migration and Health. J R Soc Med 2005;98(9):400–3.

[18] Varney H, Kriebs J, Gegor C. Varney's Midwifery 2004. 4th edition. Available at: http://books.google.com/books?id=c5dn3yh4V5UC&pg=RA1-PA64&lpg=RA1PA64&dq=essentials+of+newborn+care+immediately+after+birth&source=web&ots=h9eKnO7qJN&sig=DcgWOtX-GdG9GZ-mIlHaLp68BTU#PRA1-PA64,M1. Accessed December 30, 2007.

[19] Williams D. Giving birth "in place": a guide to emergency preparedness for childbirth J Midwifery Womens Health 2004;49(4):48–52.

[20] Centers for Disease Control and Prevention. Guidelines for vaccinating pregnant women 2007. Available at: http://www.cdc.gov/vaccines/pubs/preg-guide.htm. Accessed January 15, 2008.

[21] Cunningham FG, Leveno KJ, Bloom SL, et al. Williams obstetrics. 22nd edition. New York: McGraw Hill; 2005.

[22] Centers for Disease Control and Prevention. Critical needs for pregnant women during times of disaster for non-obstetric health care providers. 2005. Available at: http://www.bt.cdc.gov/disasters/pregnantdisasterhcp.asp. Accessed January 22, 2008.

[23] Yehunda R, Engel SM, Brand SR, et al. Trans generational effects of post traumatic stress disorder in babies of mothers exposed to the World Trade Center attacks during pregnancy. J Clin Endocrinol Metab 2005;90(7):4115–8.

[24] O'Heir J. Pregnancy and childbirth care following conflict and displacement: care for refugee women in low-resource settings. J Midwifery Womens Health 2004;49:14–8.

[25] Pascali-Bonaro D, Kroeger M. Continuous female companionship during childbirth: a crucial resource in times of stress or calm. J Midwifery Womens Health 2004;49:19–26.

[26] Centers for Disease Control and Prevention. Breastfeeding: recommendations: vaccinations. 2005. Available at: http://www.cdc.gov/breastfeeding/recommendations/vaccinations.htm. Accessed January 17, 2008.

[27] Position on infant feeding in emergencies. International Lactation Consultant Association. 2006. Available at: www.ilca.org/pubs/InfantFeeding-EmergPRpdf. Accessed January 18, 2008.

[28] Lederman SA, Rauh V, Weiss L, et al. The effects of the World Trade Center event on birth outcomes among term deliveries at three lower Manhattan hospitals. Environ Health Perspect 2004;112(17):1772–7.

[29] Al Gasseer N, Dresden E, Keeney GB, et al. Status of women and infants in complex humanitarian emergencies. J Midwifery Womens Health 2004;49:7–13.

[30] World Health Organization. HAC forum: why women and newborn health in emergencies? Department of making pregnancy safer and family and community health cluster. 2006. Available at: http://www.who.int/hac/events/Maternal_newborns.pdf. Accessed December 21, 2007.

[31] Drafts disaster management guidelines: care of the newborn. Indian Academy of Pediatrics. 2002. Available at: http://www.iapindia.org/prnCare.cfm. Accessed July 17, 2007.

[32] Ricci SS. Essentials of maternity, newborn, and women's health nursing. 2006. Available at: http://books.google.com/books?id=-qme7qNOxP0C&pg=RA2-PA342&lpg=RA2-PA342&dq=essentials+of+newborn+care+immediately+after+birth&source=web&ots=fhtMOa8IdJ&sig=5pRFB-EYK6pKubzzPc35CbTXyFs#PPP1,M1. Accessed December 20, 2007.

[33] Beck D. Ganges F, Goldman S, et al. Save the children: care of the newborn reference manual. 2004. Available at: http://www.whiteribbonalliance.org/Resources/Documents/Care%20of%20the%20Newborn_Reference%20Manual_Save%20the%20Children.pdf. Accessed December 19, 2007.

[34] Meister JC. Routine newborn care. In: case based pediatrics for medical students and residents. 2003. Chapter III 1. Available at: http://www.hawaii.edu/medicine/pediatrics/pedtext/s03c01.html. Accessed December 19, 2007.

[35] Behrman R, Butler AS, editors. Committee on understanding premature birth and assuring healthy outcomes preterm birth: causes, consequences, and prevention. Board on Health

Sciences Policy. 2007. Available at: http://books.nap.edu/openbook.php?record_id= 11622&page = 149. Accessed December 20, 2007.

[36] Davanzo R. Newborns in adverse conditions: issues, challenges, and interventions. J Midwifery Womens Health 2004;49(Suppl 1):S29–35.

[37] Hamilton P. ABC of labor care. Br Med J 1999;318:1403–6.

[38] Infant nutrition during disasters: breastfeeding and other options. American Academy of Pediatrics. 2007. Available at: http://www.aap.org/breastfeeding/PDF/InfantNutritionDisaster. pdf. Accessed December 21, 2007.

[39] Emergency preparedness: infant and young child care and feeding. Interagencies Working Group on Infant and Young Child Feeding in Emergencies/Infant Feeding Core Group. 2006. Available at: http://www.ennonline.net/pool/files/ife/ops-guidance-2-1-english-010307. pdf. Accessed December 21, 2007.

[40] U.S. Breastfeeding Committee information on infant and young children feeding in emergencies for UNICEF offices and partners. 2005. Available at: http://www.usbreastfeeding. org/Issue-Papers/Emergency.pdf. Accessed January 18, 2008.

[41] World Health Organization. Guiding principles for feeding infants and young children during emergencies. 2004. Available at: http://whqlibdoc.who.int/hq/2004/9241546069. pdf. Accessed January 18, 2008.

[42] Adhisivam B, Srinivasan S, Soudarssanane MB, et al. Feeding of infants and young children in tsunami affected villages in Pondicherry. Indian Pediatr 2006;43:724–7.

[43] White-Traut R. Providing a nurturing environment for infants in adverse situations: multisensory strategies for newborn care. J Midwifery Womens Health 2004;49:36–41, 266.

[44] Centers for Disease Control and Prevention. National vital statistics report. 2007. Available at: http://www.cdc.gov/nchs/data/nvsr/nvsr55/nvsr55_10.pdf. Accessed December 20, 2007.

[45] World Health Organization. Essential newborn care/introduction. 1993. Available at: http:// www.who.int/reproductive-health/publications/MSM_96_13/MSM_96_13_introduction.en. html. Accessed December 19, 2007.

[46] World Health Organization DoRHaRR. Thermal protection of the newborn: a practical guide (WHO/RHT/MSM/97.2). World Health Organization. Available at: http://www.who.int/ reproductive-health/publications/MSM_97_2_Thermal_protection_of_the_newborn/. Accessed September 28, 2005.

[47] Gershanik JJ. Escaping with VLBW neonates: caring for and transporting very low birth weight infants during a disaster. Pediatrics 2007;117:S365–8.

[48] Sirbaugh P, Gurwitch K, Macias C, et al. Caring for evacuated children housed in the astrodome: creation and implementation of a mobile pediatric emergency response team: regionalized caring for displaced children after a disaster. Pediatrics 2006;177: S428–38.

[49] Pediatric terrorism and disaster preparedness: a resource for pediatricians. Rockville (MD): Agency for Healthcare Research and Quality; 2006. AHRQ Publication Nos. 06(07)-0056 and 06(07)-0056-1, Available at: http://www.ahrq.gov/research/pedprep/resource.htm. Accessed January 18, 2008.

[50] Barkemeyer BM. Practicing neonatology in a blackout: the university hospital NICU in the midst of Hurricane Katrina: caring for children without power or water. Pediatrics 2006;117: S369–74.

[51] Carr KC. Disaster preparedness for mothers and babies: getting prepared. American College of Nurse Midwifes. The president's pen. 2006. Available at: http://www.midwife.org/ siteFiles/president/SO06PresidentsPen.pdf. Accessed December 19, 2007.

[52] Johnston C, Redlener I. Critical concepts for children in disasters identified by hands-on professionals: summary of issues demanding solutions before the next one. Pediatrics 2006;177: S458–60.

[53] Lobato MN, Yanni E, Hagar A, et al. Impact of Hurricane Katrina on newborn screening in Louisiana. Pediatrics 2007;120:e749–55.

[54] Ensuring maternal and child health during disaster. Save the children. 2004. Available at: http://www.healthynewborns.org/files/573_ENSURING_MATERNAL_AND_NEWBORN_emerg_relief.doc_1_11_05.pdf?PHPSESSID=32cdff80dc680c6a005e106d2784b59b. Accessed January 18, 2008.

[55] Beigi RH. Pandemic influenza and pregnancy: a call for preparedness planning. Obstet Gynecol 2007;109:1193–6.

[56] Glass RJ, Glass LM, Beyeler WE, et al. Targeted social distancing design for pandemic influenza. Sandia National Laboratories and Albuquerque Public High School, Albuquerque, New Mexico, USA. Emerg Infect Dis 2006;12(11):1671–81. Available at: http://www.cdc.gov/ncidod/EID/vol12no11/06-0255.htmcite, Accessed January 18, 2008.

[57] Allen AT, Flinn AM, Moore WF. The 81st medical group obstetrics and gynecology flight's role during Hurricane Katrina. Mil Med 2007;172:199–201.

[58] Sobieraj JA, Reyes J, Dunemn KN, et al. Modeling hospital response to mild and severe influenza pandemic scenarios under normal and expanded capacities. Mil Med 2007;172:486–90.

[59] Joint Commission on Accreditation of Healthcare Organizations. Surge hospitals: providing safe care in emergencies 2006. Available at: http://www.jointcommission.org/NR/rdonlyres/802E9DA4-AE80-4584-A205-48989C5BD684/0/surge_hospital.pdf. Accessed January 14, 2008.

[60] McLaughlin SB. Hazard vulnerability analysis. 2001. Available at: http://www.gnyha.org/23/File.aspx. Accessed January 14, 2008.

[61] U.S. Department of Homeland Security (DHS) Twin Cities Metro Region Emergency Management/Public Health. HSEEP Training Course Participant Manual. 2007.

[62] Hospital Incident Command System job action sheets. California Emergency Medical Services Authority. 2006. Available at: http://www.emsa.ca.gov/hics/job%20action%20sheets_ops.pdf. Accessed January 14, 2008.

[63] Personal and Family Emergency Preparedness Module. This course was created by the University of Minnesota's, Minnesota Emergency Readiness Education & Training (MERET) grant, the Academic Health Center's Office of Emergency Response (OER), and the Department of Emergency Management (DEM), with support from the Minnesota Department of Health. Available at: http://cpheo.sph.umn.edu/meret.

[64] National Child Traumatic Stress Network and National Center for PTSD. Psychological first aid: field operations guide. 2nd edition. 2006. Available at: http://www.ncptsd.va.gov/ncmain/ncdocs/manuals/PFA_V2.pdf. Accessed January 14, 2008.

[65] Buekens P, Xiong X, Harville E. Hurricanes and pregnancy. Birth 2006;33:91–3.

[66] Agency for Healthcare Research and Quality. Disaster planning drills and readiness assessment web conference. Rockville (MD): Agency for Healthcare Research and Quality. 2003. Available at: http://www.ahrq.gov/news/ulp/disastertele. Accessed January 15, 2008.

ELSEVIER
SAUNDERS

NURSING
CLINICS
OF NORTH AMERICA

Nurs Clin N Am 43 (2008) 469–476

From Ethics to Palliative Care:
A Community Hospital Experience

Lois R. Robley, PhD, RN

*Siegel Institute for Leadership, Ethics, and Character, Kennesaw State University,
Mailbox 5500, 1000 Chastain Road, Kennesaw, GA 30144, USA*

One of the most vulnerable and voiceless groups of patients within American hospitals and institutions today are those who are dying. Approximately 2 million people die in hospitals in the United States each year; only 24% of Americans die at home. This occurs despite the fact that greater than 70% of Americans have indicated that they wish to die in their own homes, in comfort, surrounded by those they love [1,2]. A host of social and professional changes are required before this public goal can be achieved. Among the general hospital population, 1 million have pain with only a fair (75%) chance of having that pain managed [3]. This bodes poorly for those who face death with all its attendant physical, psychologic, social, existential, and spiritual challenges. Death is a phenomenon of universality, because all of us die. Making the experience one of comfort and exquisite care ought to be the goal of every nurse and physician, respiratory therapist, and physical therapist not only for altruistic but for self-serving reasons. Improving end-of-life care benefits the common good. The goal of this article is to explain how one hospital system moved from ethical sensitivity about this issue to action.

Among the hospitalized dying, it is estimated that the following symptom burden would be realized in any given year: 342,000 patients with fatigue, 280,000 with anorexia, 244,000 with dyspnea, 232,000 with xerostomia, 208,000 with cough, 196,000 with pain, 148,000 with confusion, 148,000 with depression, 140,000 with nausea, 92,000 with insomnia, and 88,000 with vomiting [3]. Hospice is well known for its success at addressing the dying process and managing these symptoms. Lessons can be learned from hospice and applied to hospital and nursing home care, but to do that, dissemination of palliative care information needs to move expeditiously and fluidly from hospice to other institutions. More research is

E-mail address: lrobley@kennesaw.edu

needed to analyze the impact of innovative end-of-life programs and interventions on the dying in all locales. All this needs to happen so that the most vulnerable patients are cared for in a humane and rightful way.

Providers know who the dying are: patients who have chronic disease whose next exacerbation could well mean the end, patients who have cancer that is now refractory to conventional therapy, the frail elder with late-stage Alzheimer's disease, and the critically ill with multiple organ system failure. A simple question, "Would you be surprised if this patient were still alive 12 months from now," can easily be the trigger point for guiding a host of interventions to make the process of dying and death a humane and comfortable one. Interventions include making sure advance directives are in place and that they are honored, establishing comfort care orders for palliative care alongside curative treatments, redirecting team efforts to consider alternative goals for the whole person (rather than a body organ), and prescribing accordingly. Yet, in many of our institutional environments (eg, hospitals, nursing homes, assisted living), these interventions are paltry or are not put into place at all.

One of the most difficult challenges for ethics committees is wrought by the public belief in the philosophy of modern medical care. Attention to disease eradication, although scientifically noble and laudable, has left the American people with strong belief in the ability of professionals to conquer disease and death. Dying patients are given chemotherapy days before death, are tethered to ventilators, and are connected to vasopressor drips in the hours before death. Dying patients have tracheostomies and feeding tubes (percutaneous endoscopic gastrostomy [PEGs]) inserted. They and their families are told that such treatment is necessary if symptoms are to be controlled. Families are made to feel, whether by unspoken culture or through actual words, that they are responsible for decisions surrounding the dying process. The ravages of disease are fully apparent to health care professionals but are largely glossed over in the process of "maintaining hope" and treating the disease. Thus, the slippery slope of treatment for the improvement of the patient becomes futile treatment. There is no ill will or nefarious intent; it is just what happens when we are not absolutely sure about the appropriateness of our decisions at the time of reconciliation between curative treatment and futile treatment. That is why palliative care needs to be started early in the disease trajectory and intensified as dying draws near.

Large medical centers and community hospitals of all sizes struggle with these futility issues. The five large major medical centers that were included in the Study to Understand Prognoses and Preferences for Outcomes and Risks of Treatments (SUPPORT) found that 50% of dying patients lived their last days with moderate to severe pain and had do not resuscitate (DNR) orders written only 48 hours before death [4]. Death occurred within days of withdrawal of intensive medical therapy. The same phenomena hold true for smaller nonteaching institutions. The reasons for inadequate application of palliative care measures are (1) lack of professional education, (2) insufficient research, and (3) lack of positive experience and mentoring.

Palliative care

Palliative care is "both a philosophy of care and an organized, highly structured system for delivering care. The goal of palliative care is to prevent and relieve suffering and to support the best possible quality of life for patients and their families, regardless of the stage of the disease or the need for other therapies. Palliative care expands traditional disease-model medical treatments to include the goals of enhancing quality of life for patients and family members, helping with decision making, and providing opportunities for personal growth" [5].

Initiation of the program

The WellStar Health System's interest in addressing better palliative and end-of-life care began with its Ethics Committee. Similar to most hospital-based ethics committees, it is multidisciplinary and includes representative professionals from hospice and critical care, physicians and nurses, pastoral care, social services, and administration. The Ethics Committee has been pivotal: being responsible for policy and procedure related to patient rights, having experience with innumerable consults related to conflict about end-of-life issues, and having representatives on the committee who have a passion for better care of dying patients. "Talking it up" was what was done well. The five-hospital system made its first commitment to palliative care in 2003 with the employment of an end-of-life educated intensive care unit (ICU) nurse at each of the two large hospitals (one with 352 beds and another with 550 beds) to function as Critical Care Nurse Liaisons. The purpose of this role was to provide education for patients and their families in the ICU, foster communication among stakeholders, support families in the process of decision making, and educate colleagues in excellent end-of-life care [6]. With the success of this endeavor and calls for these services outside the ICU, the liaison nurses were later assigned to the hospice and palliative care program. In May of 2004, the system sent a team of four professionals to Mt. Carmel Hospital in Columbus, Ohio, one of the palliative care leadership centers that is similar in structure and size to the WellStar Health System. This site exemplifies excellence in palliative and end-of-life care and is authorized as a leadership center under the auspices of the Center to Advance Palliative Care (CAPC). The most important lesson learned from the visit was the importance of making the financial case for improved palliative care within one's own institution.

Along with the CAPC, a host of prominent professional organizations, including the American Association of Colleges of Nursing and the American College of Surgeons, endorsed the National Quality Forum (NQF) clinical practice guidelines [7]. These guidelines address quality palliative care, including the following aspects of care: (1) structure and processes; (2) physical; (3) psychologic and psychiatric; (4) social; (5) spiritual, religious, and existential; (6) cultural; (7) care of the imminently dying; and (8) ethical and legal. The NQF endorses preferred clinical practices that should serve to guide the improvement of hospice and palliative care across the nation.

The WellStar Health System addressed several areas for improvement using the knowledge gained from the CAPC, historical and clinical experience, the Joint Commission for the Accreditation of Health Care Organizations (JCAHO) standards for end-of-life and patient rights, and benchmarks identified in the professional literature. These included advance directives, refusal of care, individual cultural needs, reassessing pain management, and patient rights. The system sought to achieve consistent end-of-life standards and maximize reimbursement using ethical guidelines across various delivery sites: the hospitals, nursing home, long-term care center, home health care, and residential and home hospice. The principles of respect for others—caring, justice, and beneficence—were used as guidelines for decision making.

The Ethics Committee was systematically involved in readiness planning for a possible flu pandemic. A document for ethical conduct of triage and assisting with the care of the dying during a pandemic that was developed out of the Ethics Center at Emory University was used to guide policy development and action [8]. Also, in 2005, data were gathered about the number of deaths within the system, excluding those that were trauma induced and those in hospice and home health. Approximately 1000 deaths occurred that year, which gave system administrators a sense of the scope of the problem. Attention was drawn to the plight of the dying, and programs were intensified to honor the autonomy of patients and support patients and families through end-of-life decision making.

Phase 1

More education was needed for the entire professional staff, with the goal of baseline knowledge of palliative care for all, alongside expert consultation. The first step was to address advanced directives. Newly employed staff and existing employees in nursing learned how to determine, acknowledge, respect, and honor advance directives through didactic and on-line education [9]. An inpatient admission packet was developed to instruct patients and their families; the admitting nurse now initials the chart when those materials are provided and discussed. Any patient requesting more information about advance directives is directed to one uniform resource: social services. In the largest of the WellStar Health System's hospitals, a social worker was hired to handle all advance directive issues, educating and advocating for patients. The Critical Care Nurse Liaisons were also pivotal in educating staff, patients, and families about advance directives. Education was conducted by the physician/chairperson of the Ethics Committee at the system's yearly Ethics Forum for several years running. At meetings of nursing leadership, advance directives, updates on patient rights, and the developing palliative care program were explained. Interdisciplinary end-of-life education was begun, using End of Life Nursing Education Consortium (ELNEC) materials presented by a facilitator/trainer for registered nurses and discharge planners [10]. A community member of the Ethics Committee conducted Ethics Rounds monthly that addressed bedside ethics dilemmas, most of which have to do with end-of-life issues. Story boards were developed and displayed in key locations for employees and were included in skills days for nurses. Nurses were educated regarding the JCAHO criteria, taught to document advance directives on the chart, and informed about the process of honoring advance directives as dictated by Georgia law. Physicians were encouraged to solicit advance directives in their practice by the Ethics Committee chairperson at medical staff meetings.

Phase 2

Most crucial to problem solving in individual cases was the need for palliative care to be made visible to physicians who were blinded for years by their lack of education about palliation and their indentured attitude of disease eradication. A more holistic view of the person, rather than the disease entity, needed to be engendered, and it was acknowledged that this would take personal contact. This move started with a simple change in titles. In 2005, the position of Critical Care Nurse Liaison was newly titled Palliative Care Liaison and moved from the Ethics Committee to reside under hospice and palliative care. Services were made available beyond critical care to the entire inpatient population, and symptom management was the goal. Hospice algorithms are used for making recommendations to physicians for symptom management and medications. Evidence-based practice was employed to use nonpharmacologic comfort measures, including emotional and spiritual care that incorporates pastoral care for both purposes. Bereavement programs are currently being expanded from within hospice, to include hospitalized patients in palliative care and also to those bereaved within the community. Hospital chaplains, along with community clergy, work closely with the Palliative Care Liaison nurses. New order sets were developed for withdrawal from the ventilator and comfort care. These new policies wended their way through the approval process piloted by nurses and doctors from within the Ethics Committee and hospice. A separate position was also created for a registered nurse to assess for hospice eligibility within the hospitals. The CAPC financial formulas were used with the WellStar hospital information to take a unique look at the savings that could be realized as inpatient days are reduced. To aid in the transition of palliative to acute care, four to six hospital beds have been assigned as palliative care beds, and the average length of stay is 4 days with transfer to home hospice, residential hospice, or a nursing home with hospice oversight.

Phase 3

In 2006, recruitment was launched to hire a full-time palliative care physician. This process took 18 months, and as of January, 2008, the system has a board-certified hospice and palliative care physician available to guide excellence of palliative care. Simultaneously, the Ethics Committee chairperson was on an educational mission to inform physicians regarding palliative care: to prepare them for the hospital multidisciplinary team approach to palliative care and understand the newly created division for palliative care. The electronic medical record was begun for hospice care, which should facilitate communication among entities within the system.

Also in 2006, the Dartmouth Atlas of Health Care [11] (Wennberg and colleagues, 2006) report was published. It demonstrated that the chronically ill and dying of America who are hospitalized in the last 6 months of their lives do not have better, and may even have worse, health outcomes than those cared for in their communities. Also, it was shown that the states and regions vary significantly in their use of Medicare dollars for the dying, with little or no significant difference in outcomes. Benchmarking and a move to less costly and less intensive care for the chronically ill are advocated.

In keeping with these trends, the focus of activity in 2007 was on decreasing hospital mortality. Most people wish to die at home surrounded by the familiar environment and loved ones; thus, the Wellstar Health System's passion is to help achieve that goal. The revised law in Georgia regarding advance directives gives added impetus: it directly states to physicians that if the provisions of the advance directives are contrary to the beliefs and practices of the individual physician, the patient's care is to be transferred to a physician who can honor the wishes of the patient. This revision of the law assists with education and helps to support the efforts of those who are interested in preventing conflict and making the system respectful of patient's considered and enduring wishes.

Evaluation

Early in 2007, focus groups were conducted with physicians and nurses within the system to learn about their knowledge of advance directives and end-of-life care. Taking the perspective that going back to square one and addressing poor outcomes and lack of information often spur change, the findings have been useful to the process of education. It was discovered that the staff were unfamiliar with the legal parameters related to end-of-life care and advance directives. There was a significant gulf between the perception of the dying patient and her or his needs on the part of physicians and nurses. These perceptions seem to hark back to differences in education and their understanding of the professional role in treatment decisions for the whole patient. As Byock [12] says about medical education: "required training in communication, pain assessment and management, ethics of decision-making and guidance for people facing life's end is scant and has increased only marginally in recent years. Most graduating students and licensed physicians have never been taught to assess and treat cancer pain, know little about hospice care and have not been trained in ways to counsel a person with advanced illness who worries about the future or has begun to feel that life is not worth living. Today's young doctors are bright, caring, committed and generally well-trained professionals, but they weren't born with the aforementioned skills, nor have they been taught them." Likewise, in nursing, end-of-life education has been lacking. Coyle [13] quotes a nurse saying "I failed to care for him properly because I was ignorant...the memory haunts me." This might be said by thousands of nurses whose formal nursing education, even today, lacks sufficient information about end-of-life care.

Next steps

Education throughout the system and jointly among all disciplines about palliative care remains an essential goal of the Ethics Committee. Ethics week presentations, one-on-one education of all staff, Ethics Rounds, and formal education at regularly scheduled meetings of staff are staples of educational programming. It is in the everyday encounters and all relationships among professionals that progress is going to be made. Diligence and modeling are important for the palliative care team. In the future, it is hoped that end-of-life volunteers can be employed to assist patients and families navigate the system, learn about excellent end-of-life care, and provide presence and support. The hypothesis is that with more education on palliative care and greater consultation and dialog by physicians with the palliative care team, fewer ethics consults are likely to be required. In effect, prevention of conflict would be realized.

Acknowledgments

The author thanks Dr. Richard Cohen, Chairperson of the WellStar Ethics Committee, and Charlene Bunts, Director of WellStar Palliative Care and Hospice, for their assistance with this article.

References

[1] Field M, Cassell C. Approaching death: improving care at the end of life. Committee on Care at the End of Life, Institute of Medicine. Washington, DC: National Academy Press; 1997.
[2] The Center for Gerontology and Health Care Research. Facts on dying: policy relevant data on care at the end of life. Brown University. Available at: http://www.chcr.brown.edu/dying/USASTATISTICS.HTM. Published 2006. Accessed January 10, 2008.
[3] Von Gunten CF. Interventions to manage symptoms at the end of life. J Palliat Med 2005; 8(Suppl 1):S88–94.

[4] Desbiens NA, Wu AW, Broste SK, et al. Pain and satisfaction with pain control in seriously ill hospitalized adults: findings from the SUPPORT research investigations. Crit Care Med 1996;24:S88–S94.

[5] Ferrell BR, Connor SR, Cordes A, et al. The national agenda for quality palliative care: the national consensus project and the national quality forum. J Pain Symptom Manage 2007; 33:737–44.

[6] Robley L, Denton S. Evaluation of an EOL critical care nurse liaison program. Journal of Hospice & Palliative Nursing 2006;8:288–93.

[7] National Quality Forum. Clinical practice guidelines for quality palliative care. National Consensus Project. Available at: http://www.qualityforum.org/publications/reports/palliative.asp. Published 2007. Accessed January 10, 2008.

[8] Kinlaw K, Levine R. Ethical guidelines in pandemic influenza. Recommendations of the Ethics Subcommittee of the Advisory Committee to the Director, Centers for Disease Control and Prevention. February 15, 2007.

[9] Bakitas MA. Self-determination: analysis of the concept and implications for research in palliative care. Can J Nurs Res 2005;37:22–49.

[10] American Association of Colleges of Nursing. End-of-life Nursing Education Consortium (ELNEC) Web site. Available at: http://www.aacn.nche.edu/ELNEC/. Accessed January 10, 2007.

[11] McAndrew M, Bronner KK. The care of patients with severe chronic illness: an online report on the Medicare program by the Dartmouth Atlas Project. Dartmouth Medical Center. Available at: http://www.dartmouthatlas.org/atlases/2006_Chronic_Care_Atlas.pdf. Published 2006. Accessed January 10, 2008.

[12] Byock I. House Human Services Committee testimony on House Bill 44. March 1, 2007:1–2.

[13] Coyle N. Introduction to palliative care nursing. In: Ferrell BR, Coyle N, editors. Textbook of palliative nursing. 2nd edition. New York: Oxford University Press; 2006. p. 2–11.

NURSING
CLINICS
OF NORTH AMERICA

Nurs Clin N Am 43 (2008) 477–489

Vulnerable Populations:
Drug Court Program Clients

Patricia M. Speck, DNSc, FNP-BC, FAAN,
FAAFS, DF-IAFN, SANE-A, SANE-P[a],*,
Pamela D. Connor, PhD[b],
Margaret T. Hartig, PhD, PFNP, FNP-BC[a],
Patricia D. Cunningham, DNSc, APRN-PMH,
FNP-BC[a], Belinda Fleming, PhD(c), MSN, FNP-BC[a]

[a]College of Nursing, The University of Tennessee Health Science Center, 877 Madison
Avenue, Lamar Alexander Building, 6th Floor, Memphis, TN 38163, USA
[b]Department of Preventive Medicine, College of Medicine, The University of Tennessee
Health Science Center, 66 N. Pauline Street, 6th Floor, Memphis, TN 38163, USA

Case study

Maria was married with children and gainfully employed before she became a breast cancer survivor. She was given several medications for pain and became addicted. Her husband left her after a "huge fight," in which he beat her and took the children. She was diagnosed with depression unable to support herself; eventually, she lost her job and became homeless before landing in drug court with a charge of prostitution. Her boyfriend wants her to take the sentence and get out of the drug court program.

Discussion points:

1. Enrollees may want to recover but may not have the resources to leave a lifestyle.
2. Skills for employment are necessary for sustaining recovery.
3. Hope of regaining a relationship with children may be a motivator for recovery.
4. History of violence or homelessness may impede recovery if not addressed.

———————
Grant funding for health and risk assessments provided by State of Tennessee Office of Justice Programs to the Shelby County Drug Court (SCDC) and the SCDC Support Foundation.

* Corresponding author. The University of Tennessee Health Science Center, College of Nursing, 877 Madison Avenue, Room 653, Memphis, TN 38163.

E-mail address: pspeck@utmem.edu (P.M. Speck).

5. Mental health diagnoses may reduce compliance with program goals.

Incarceration and drug use statistics

It is predicted that 2.3 million persons would be incarcerated in the United States in 2006 [1]. A significant number of these individuals have mental health problems and also are without health care and support services in the community [2]. Arrest for drug use, misuse, addiction, mental illnesses, and sale of drugs become reasons for incarceration, resulting in drug offenders[1] making up a large percentage of inmates. The explanations for the vulnerability associated with the drug offender's incarceration are multifaceted and complex. Some believe that society's zeal to incarcerate drug offenses resulted in "ineffective" and "cruel" punishment in addition to a significant outlay of precious financial resources [3,4]. Others encourage strict sentencing for criminals convicted of committing crimes without regard for the underlying use, abuse, and addiction issues facing the individual [4]. The communities that enacted mandatory sentencing soon realized that the criminal would be released and that most would relapse and reoffend by repeating the same crimes—all attributable to drug-seeking behavior [5–8]. The "Just Say No" campaign of the 1980s did not work [9]. Prisons remain overcrowded today with vulnerable populations that are (1) convicted of crimes associated with drug use, (2) unemployable (eg, ex-convict, no skills or education), (3) uninsured because they are unemployed, and (4) in need of treatment for their addictions and mental illnesses, childhood emotional traumas, and the physical health sequelae from an at-risk lifestyle while using drugs [8,10–18]. Another approach was needed to slow this movement toward long sentences in incarceration of drug offenders and their addictions. The additional impact on families, the offender's children, and communities has reached a crisis stage for those who are entangled in the criminal justice system, making drug offenders the largest number of inmates in prisons [19,20].

Another model was needed to slow this movement toward long sentences in incarceration of drug offenders and their addictions. Responding to these pressures in the late 1980s, the Robert Wood Johnson Foundation funded an experimental project in the court of Miami Dade County, Florida to address the treatment needs of this vulnerable population caught in the criminal justice system because they were "drug offenders" [21]. This project became the model for current drug court programs and their interventions.

Introduction to drug court

Since the first drug court in Miami, Dade County, Florida, drug courts have demonstrated success in the treatment of drug-related disorders. An

---

[1] Definition: Human Rights Watch defines "'Drug' offenders are prisoners admitted with a drug offense (e.g., possession, using or selling) as their most serious offense. Anyone convicted of both a crime of violence and a drug offense would be categorized as a violent offender" [4].

additional advantage is cost reduction for the criminal justice system by keeping the drug user out of jail. The number of programs has grown to "over 2,000 in over 1,100 counties" across the United States in 2007 [22,23]. The function and role of the drug court have not changed in nearly 2 decades, but evidence is building to help understand the nuances of why an individual responds positively to the program. As a diversionary program, drug court is an alternative to jail; as a treatment program, the addiction is seen as disease requiring medical intervention [24,25]. Combined, the focused efforts and coordinated supervision throughout the phases of recovery using the drug court procedures create a level of accountability not seen in traditional methods of addressing crimes related to drug misuse [26].

Key components of the drug court program must be present to be certified or become a mentor court. Additionally, those involved must be willing to train others who want to duplicate the activities [27]. These components include integration of treatment services into the case processing of the court, use of a "nonadversarial" approach toward the criminal justice professionals, the early identification and placement of clients, access to treatment and rehabilitation, monitored abstinence and compliance programs, ongoing interaction with the clients enrolled in the program through monitoring achievement of program goals, interdisciplinary education to promote effective operations, and development of partnerships with community-based organizations that ensure the drug court program's effectiveness [26].

These components are necessary because drug courts seek to assist in the recovery of the client. Accountability is core to the process. Close supervision and surveillance may include frequent activities, such as reporting to the court and urine tests for drugs or consequences for noncompliance with the strict rules [3,24,26]. Consequences vary from the offender returning to transitional and supervised housing to requiring additional jail time or court appearances for infractions of the rules. These sanctions place considerable stress on the clients when they are separated from their communities, jobs, families, and especially their children [3,21,28]. Serious infractions may result in expulsion from the program. Ultimately, those expelled may be subject to significant incarceration for the crime(s) committed before entering the drug court program [8,10,13,29–31].

The drug court process is relatively simple, beginning with the choice to participate after an arrest for a drug-related nonviolent crime. The offender petitions the court for acceptance into the program and enters a guilty plea to the charges, usually in response to knowledge that there is significant jail time if convicted in a regular court. This plea[2] is held while the offender is enrolled in the drug court program. The enrollee then follows the regimen of close supervision through three or four phases of recovery. If the offender

---

[2] "Plea in abeyance" is the legal term for a guilty plea and is held until successful completion of the program when it will be withdrawn.

violates the terms and reoffends or uses, he or she faces sentencing and imprisonment. If he or she successfully completes the phases of recovery, he or she has the guilty plea withdrawn and the charges are dismissed.

Phases of recovery are defined by the level of supervision and may vary among drug courts. The following is an example of the drug court phases in the first program in the nation. The Miami, Dade County, Florida Drug Court program has three phases, with drug testing and monitoring throughout the entire program. They include the following:

Phase I: Detoxification (12–15 days but often continues longer when clients have difficulty getting off drugs). Once clients have volunteered to enter the program, they are transferred to the county's main treatment clinic to begin detoxification. During this time, the counselor and client work together to prepare a treatment plan that sets realistic short- and long-term goals, identifies barriers to achieving these goals, and develops strategies to overcome obstacles. Treatment includes group and individual counseling, 12-step fellowship meetings, and inpatient treatment, if necessary. Approximately 85% of drug court participants also use acupuncture to reduce withdrawal symptoms. Counselors recommend that clients move on to phase II based on an overall impression of their ability to succeed in a less restrictive environment. At minimum, they must have attended all 12 scheduled sessions with their primary counselor and have at least seven consecutive clean urine results.

Phase II: Stabilization (14–16 weeks but can vary from 2 months to more than a year). In the second phase, clients concentrate on keeping clean by attending individual and group counseling sessions and fellowship meetings, and they often continue acupuncture treatments. As in every phase, counselors allow clients to decide on the types of treatment as long as their urine tests remain negative and they attend required treatment and court sessions.

Phase III: Aftercare (8–9 months but may be longer depending on the individual's ability to stay drug free). Treatment continues in phase III, but clients also begin preparing for the future by developing educational and vocational skills for successful re-entry into the community. This may include literacy and general equivalency diplomat (GED) classes, financial aid, employability skills, and training and job development classes in addition to access to current job listings and training programs [32].

Case study

Corey was a 22-year-old high-school dropout who was arrested because he was a passenger in a vehicle with a person in possession of marijuana. He initially denied a habit but eventually admitted to smoking "weed" since he was 10 years old. He now reports that he no longer smokes marijuana but that he still has friends who do. He was released from "24/7" transitional housing, in which he had been undergoing treatment for his addiction and vocational training for the past 6 months. After a holiday weekend, he tested positive for marijuana again but denies that he used. He did report that his parents were smoking marijuana all weekend and the house was full of the smoke. He was sent back to jail for 3 days to think about it.

Discussion points:

1. Family members who use illicit drugs pose additional burdens on the person in treatment.
2. Enrollees who depend on family for housing need help to find housing away from those who could ultimately result in the enrollee receiving maximum time in jail.
3. The community of systems failed this young man in the identification of illicit drug use in his family, from which he might have been removed.
4. Buffering the addict from those who put the enrollee at risk is foundational to recovery.
5. Changing belief systems is foundational for treatment to be effective.
6. Education, whether vocational or GED, is valuable to conduct personal business.
7. Training for a job and employment are important for success and graduation from the program.

Many courts partner with community organizations to improve educational achievement. The client may be re-enrolled in the GED program that awards a diploma [33,34]. In Memphis, Tennessee, the drug court offered its first scholarship for an enrollee who aspired to graduate from college in 2007. Preparing the enrollee for employment, along with readiness to participate, is an important component of a comprehensive approach to the client who is struggling to complete the program. As courts strive to retain clients in the program, lessons can be learned from working with other vulnerable populations.

The drug court client

The drug court client is primarily African American and male. Disparities in sentencing have been clearly identified for African Americans, creating a population of men and women who are disproportionately charged and incarcerated for drug-related crimes [4]. Addiction occurs when one compulsively searches for a substance, even when he or she knows its use has harmful sequelae to himself, herself, or families [35]. Although the first uses of drugs are voluntary, eventually, the brain changes in structure and function, making it difficult to seek treatment and stop using the drug; for some, it can also cloud judgment, wherein the individual may make decisions that are not in his or her personal best interest [35]. The evidence supports the belief that addiction is like a chronic disease, in which providers have learned to expect relapses throughout the course of the disease; today, providers plan for new treatments that address the relapses in the course of the disease [35].

The disease of addiction creates chaos that prevents health-seeking behaviors. As a result, adults rarely report their first experiment with drugs or alcohol in adulthood. The vulnerability to drug use can begin in adolescence or childhood, and the youngest are more vulnerable to addiction [35]. In addition, "adolescents who smoke, drink and/or use drugs have poorer health, more health problems, and more hospitalizations than adolescents who abstain from these behaviors" [36]. Some believe that adolescents use illicit drugs to mask mental health problems, such as depression and suicide, aggression or violence, or personality disorders [36,37]. These comorbid medical and mental health conditions of the adolescent's high-risk lifestyle carry over into adulthood and, with the chaotic at-risk lifestyle of the drug user (ie, drug delivery systems [needles or smoking], or sexual intercourse [ie, with hundreds of partners]), may result in exposure to diseases such as hepatitis C, HIV, other subclinical sexually transmitted infections (STIs); respiratory illnesses; and heart or vessel disease [38]. Consequently, the use of and addiction to drugs and alcohol create a burden on the health care system when unattended infections turn into abscesses requiring surgery, cancers are undetected in early stages, chronic disease is untreated, and a crash or other injury results in serious and sudden use of emergency health care systems [38].

Although some enrolled in drug courts are members of a population considered statistically more vulnerable (ie, African American), responses from drug court clients in Memphis about the use of health care systems during their periods of drug use resulted in the coining of a new term to describe this population: "never served" [38]. In other words, the patient who is in need of basic preventative health services not only does not use the health care system, but he or she does not want treatment for the drug use and abuse [38,39]. By this definition, the never-served populations who opt out of traditional health care services and are missed in traditional health care data collection systems also include the homeless, at risk young to middle-aged males, victims of domestic violence and rape, other addicted users, and drug court populations [3,21,38,40]. These individuals are only identified by the health care system when they arrive amenable to treatment with a serious life-threatening illness or injury for care that is complicated by attitudes and beliefs of youth and the comorbidities of unstable mental disorders and long-term and life-threatening medical disease [31,39,41].

Vulnerability in the drug court population

As evidence mounts as to what interventions work, the successes of individuals enrolled in drug court programs improve. After nearly 2 decades, it is clear that the drug court alternative of jail (incarceration) is expensive, punitive, and does not help families or communities to improve quality of life. When the population of drug court enrollees is compared with those who are jailed for their drug-related offenses, approximately 70% of the drug court participant cohort graduate from the program, secure jobs, return to their families, and become productive sober citizens. The recidivism rate for the drug court graduates is only 17%, compared with the 66% of those who are incarcerated and not treated [22].

The ripple effect of the drug court clients' sentencing touches multiple systems and has an impact on individuals, families and children, and the communities in which they reside. This population meets the definition of vulnerable as described by Sebastian [40] in Stanhope and Lancaster's *Public Health Nursing*: "...a subgroup of the population that is more likely to develop health problems as a result of exposure to risk or to have worse outcomes from these health problems than the rest of the population."

The risk marker for this population is drug court enrollment, a factor associated with a higher prevalence of medical and mental health diseases [38,40,42,43]. Although there are health disparities among the members of the population of drug court clients, these disparities center around race [28,44], geography (rural and urban) [39], employment [11,12], and mental health access to care [2,36]. The drug court population, however, also meets the criteria for disadvantaged [41] in that on arrest, they have fewer resources with which to receive treatment for the myriad of health care needs for themselves and their families [4,5,10,28,31,38,40,43].

The health status of the clients enrolled in the drug court program has not been evaluated in depth even though key component 4 mandates that drug courts "provide access to a continuum of treatment and rehabilitation services" [26]. Although it is suspected that the drug court population's health mirrors the prison population's health, it is not known what health disparities exist in access to care, quality of care, or health outcomes in this cohort. The Institute of Medicine's (IOM) [45] definition of disparity is "racial or ethnic related factors or clinical needs, preferences, and appropriateness of intervention." Although this population cohort is not identified as ethnic or racial, it is suggested that the drug court enrollee who is a member of an identified group is affected disproportionately by health disparities; others may be included, because the members of the cohort report that they do not trust systems and do not seek out the establishment for health care. Historically, attitudes by health care providers that stereotype the addict who has committed crimes result in prejudice toward the addict and ex-convict, which are criteria for experiencing health disparities. In addition, the unemployed addict who is mandated to transitional housing and court appearances is generally not insured and experiences fragmented health care [38], all identified by the IOM as components of health disparities [45], in which social and political factors play a large part in the acceptance of the drug court enrollee back into society [41]. Arguably, this population is vulnerable, and as a demographic subpopulation, they experience health disparities that demand inclusion as a targeted group. *Healthy People 2010* [46] responded and now includes persons in groups characterized by their disability, but in the description of what constitutes a disability, the drug user or addict is not included.

Health Evaluation and Lifestyle Promotion (HELP) Center findings

Understanding the dynamics of a high-risk lifestyle in the drug court population, a pilot health screening evaluation was undertaken by the University of Tennessee Health Science Center, College of Nursing, to implement key component 4 and discover the extent of illness and injury in this population [38]. Volunteers were referred from the drug court and answered questions about their drug use experiences and feelings about themselves, their lifestyle, and their health. The sample nearly reflected the racial breakdown in the greater Memphis area of 62% African American, 36% white, and 2% Asian. There were 42% female and 58% male volunteers. The population was split into two groups divided by the ages of younger than 29 years (44%) and older than 30 years (56%), ranging from 18 to 58 years of age. They were all evaluated for health history, exposure to risk, mental health, and current physical health status. The results of the evaluation revealed multiple at-risk lifestyle behaviors related to health, including smoking (82%); obesity (85%), in which clients gained weight after drug court enrollment; and multiple sexual partners, with some reporting more than 100. Dental disease was discovered in 73% of the sample and included dental caries and discoloration from drug use, broken teeth from neglect and injury, temporary fillings, and abscesses in the broken teeth. Thirty-nine (39%) individuals were discovered to have hepatitis B or C with resulting liver disease (17%) and hypercholesterolemia (54%). The smokers had respiratory disease (32%), ear pathologic conditions (50%), and cardiovascular pathologic conditions (33%). Those with multiple sexual partners had genitourinary diseases (43%) and asymptomatic STIs (17%). Many reported that they had experienced deadly intrafamilial violence of a first, or second-degree relative (25%). Fifty-four percent (54%) had been diagnosed with a mental health problem, but few took the medicine prescribed because they had no money or benefits and they were consumed by addictive behaviors. A portion of the sample reported that they had received no health care in 5 or more years (32%), and another 22% reported that they had never been seen by a health care provider. Fully half of the volunteer sample was never served by the health care community. The myth is that drug users are receiving government assistance to support their habit, but only 8% of this sample sought government assistance and it was for their children. White men were most vulnerable to using more types of drugs than all other groups [38].

It was clear after this pilot study that this population is in dire need of health care because they are disadvantaged and have fewer resources (eg, no job, no supportive family, many have no hope), have overall poor health after a high-risk lifestyle, and lack the health care resources to seek providers who are willing to work with the complex issues facing recovering addicts, especially while tethered to drug court programs and mandatory transitional housing. As a result of these findings, nursing efforts to partner with community providers have met with some success, especially the partnerships with the local health department and clinic for the "working poor." Once the enrollee has successfully completed the first two phases of recovery and the court's phased schedule allows for gainful employment, the sober clients begin to take care of themselves. If the teeth were marred, broken, or infected, it is not unusual to see the first self-care intervention being oral health care [38]. If the job offers insurance, the client signs up. Vocalized desires to "get well" are common. The efforts made demonstrate that the recovering addict does make decisions that are in his or her best interest. Barriers remain, however, for those with active hepatitis C, because the treatment is too expensive and, for them, not available at this time.

The system's response

The drug court enrollee is in a restorative environment throughout the phased recovery. The environment of the criminal justice system (eg, social and support services) and the community partners (eg, primary mental health care) provides a team approach to therapeutic case management focusing on the unique characteristics of the individual enrollee. Although the fourth key component recommends access to primary health care [26], outside the jail health screening (eg, tuberculosis [TB], STI, HIV), many communities have not provided the medical care necessary for comprehensive services [38,43]. Health care providers have not been willing to embrace this population either. Their needs for health and mental health care are complex and require multidisciplinary and interprofessional approaches to break down the barriers that prevent re-entry of the recovered addict into society [3,45]. The absence of systems that provide outreach for health and social resources creates a window of opportunity for public health, forensic, and advanced practice nurses wanting to develop comprehensive services[3] for the drug court client until employment affords the sober graduate health insurance options, removing one barrier to access to care.

Comprehensive services for the newly enrolled drug court client should provide several services that address their immediate medical health and mental health needs. These health care services would include treatment of infections (eg, STIs), upper respiratory infections, or irritating skin lesions from "picking" and diagnosis of mental health problems. Psychologic triage and medical treatment at the time of arrest could prevent the

---

[3] Comprehensive services are health services that focus on more than one health problem or concern [40].

potentially life-threatening detoxification of the inmate during the initial incarceration. Health promotion and prevention services could provide educational materials to the clients that improve health by targeting specific behaviors (eg, smoking, healthy eating habits, addiction). Comprehensive evaluation by safety-net providers[4] could identify self-limiting and chronic diseases for which treatments could and should be initiated and progress toward a healthier lifestyle monitored until a permanent primary care provider is located. Finally, when patients have serious medical needs (ie, diabetic ketosis; pneumonia, kidney, or liver failure), a partnership with the walk-in emergency department would provide access to urgent care and a pathway to hospitalization. These efforts, combined with the efforts of the drug court team of criminal justice professionals and treatment providers, envelop the client with therapeutic support and accountability.

The restorative approach to provide comprehensive health care for this vulnerable population of drug court clients meets the key component recommendations to consider primary medical problems, including HIV and STIs. Public health nurses should continue to examine and challenge attitudes and beliefs about the health of addicts and drug users by scrutinizing policy decisions about the evidence to support priorities that result in social justice through treatment modalities for the recovering addict. The public health nurse should serve on local boards to influence community attitudes and services directed toward the recovering user who is also involved in petty crime. Knowledge about the court's primary interest is important, realizing that the drug court client is complex and there are several other situations that should be addressed with the user during the recovery phases as well. They include homelessness, intimate partner violence, childhood experiences (eg, sexual abuse), and unemployment, to name a few.

Because dollars are scarce and transitional housing and medical and mental health treatment are limited, relapses should be expected and interventions should be planned for this inevitable outcome. Choosing the right interventions to work for the individual drug court client should dominate the daily work of the drug court team. The addicted vulnerable and disadvantaged cannot be served in their local community, however, until drug courts can operate at full capacity, providing comprehensive health and mental health care by serving all who are eligible for this important program.

Acknowledgments

This article was written and edited primarily by Dr. Speck. Drs. Connor, Hartig, and Cunningham and B. Fleming provided content expertise, added significant information in their content areas, and edited the document.

---

[4] Safety net providers "increase access to health and social services for vulnerable populations with limited financial ability to pay for care" [47].

References

[1] Fellner J. US addiction to incarceration puts 2.3 million in prison. Human Rights News. December 1, 2006. Available at: http://hrw.org/english/docs/2006/12/01/usdom14728.htm. Accessed January 3, 2008.

[2] Tyuse SW, Linhorst DM. Drug courts and mental health courts: implications for social work [Journal Peer Reviewed Journal]. Health Soc Work 2005;30(3):233–40.

[3] Cooper CS. Drug courts—just the beginning: getting other areas of public policy in sync [Journal Peer Reviewed Journal]. Subst Use Misuse 2007;42(2–3):243–56.

[4] Fellner J, Walsh S, Roth K, et al. Punishment and prejudice: racial disparities in the war on drugs. 2000. Available at: http://www.hrw.org/reports/2000/usa/. Accessed January 2, 2008.

[5] Fielding JE, Tye G, Ogawa PL, et al. Los Angeles County drug court programs: initial results. J Subst Abuse Treat 2002;23(3):217–24.

[6] Hannett MJ. Lessening the sting of ASFA: the rehabilitation-relapse dilemma brought about by drug addiction and termination of parental rights [Journal Peer Reviewed Journal]. Family Court Review 2007;45(3):524–37.

[7] Hepburn JR, Harvey AN. The effect of the threat of legal sanction on program retention and completion: is that why they stay in drug court? [Journal Peer Reviewed Journal] Crime Delinq 2007;53(2):255–80.

[8] Webster J, Rosen PJ, McDonald HS, et al. Mental health as a mediator of gender differences in employment barriers among drug abusers [Journal Peer Reviewed Journal]. Am J Drug Alcohol Abuse 2007;33(2):259–65.

[9] Elliott J. Just say nonsense—Nancy Reagan's drug education programs. Washington Monthly. Available at: http://findarticles.com/p/articles/mi_m1316/is_n5_v25/ai_13786316/pg_1. Accessed January 1–3, 2008.

[10] Janikowski WR, Afflitto FM, Morrozoff DL, et al. Process evaluation of the Shelby County Drug Court (Process evaluation) Memphis (TN): University of Memphis. 2000.

[11] Leukefeld C, McDonald HS, Staton M, et al. Employment, employment-related problems, and drug use at drug court entry [Journal Peer Reviewed Journal]. Subst Use Misuse 2004; 39(13–14):2559–79.

[12] Leukefeld C, Webster J, Staton-Tindall M, et al. Employment and work among drug court clients: 12-month outcomes [Journal Peer Reviewed Journal]. Subst Use Misuse 2007;42(7): 1109–26.

[13] Roll JM, Prendergast M, Richardson K, et al. Identifying predictors of treatment outcome in a drug court program [Journal Peer Reviewed Journal]. Am J Drug Alcohol Abuse 2005; 31(4):641–56.

[14] Kemp K, Savitz B, Thompson W, et al. Developing employment services for criminal justice clients enrolled in drug user treatment programs. Substance Use & Misuse 2004;39(13–4): 2491–511.

[15] Greenberg GA, Rosenheck RA. Jail incarceration, homelessness, and mental health: a national study. Psychiatric Services 2008;59(2):170–7.

[16] Freudenberg N, Daniels J, Crum M, et al. Coming home from jail: the social and health consequences of community reentry for women, male adolescents, and their families and communities. American Journal of Public Health 2005;95(10):1725–36.

[17] Zannis DA, Savitz B, Thompson W, et al. Predictors of criminal recidivism 24 months following parole. Journal of Drug Issues 2003;33(1):223–36.

[18] Zink T. Hamilton County Family Treatment Drug Court. Rochester (MN): Olmsted Medical Center; 2006.

[19] Blumstein A, Beck A. Population growth in U.S. prisons, 1980–1996. In: Tonry M, Petersilia J, editors. Prisons. Chicago: University of Chicago Press; 1999. p. 17–62.

[20] Field GD. Historical trends of drug treatment in the criminal justice system. In: Leukefeld CG, Timms F, Farabee D, editors. Treatment of drug offenders: policies and issues. New York: Springer; 2002. p. 9–21.

[21] Cooper CS. Drug courts: current issues and future perspectives. Subst Use Misuse 2003; 38(11–13):1671–711.

[22] Huddleston CW, Freeman-Wilson K, Boone D. Painting the current picture: a national report card on drug courts and other problem solving court programs in the United States. Available at: www.ndci.org/publications/paintingcurrentpicture.pdf. Accessed January 1–3, 2008.

[23] Unze D. Drug courts offer offenders alternatives. USA Today 2007. Available at: http:// www.usatoday.com/news/nation/2007-12-20-alternativecourts_N.htm. Accessed January 1–3, 2008.

[24] National Institute of Justice. Drug courts: the second decade. 2006. Available at: www.ncjrs. gov/pdffiles1/nij/211081.pdf. Accessed January 1–3, 2008.

[25] Office of Justice Programs. Looking at a decade of drug courts. 1998. Available at: http:// www.ncjrs.gov/html/bja/decade98.htm. Accessed January 1–3, 2008.

[26] National Institute of Justice. Defining drug courts: the key components. Retrieved. 1997. Available at: www.nadcp.org/docs/dkeypdf.pdf. Accessed January 1–3, 2008.

[27] Office of Criminal Justice Programs. Tennessee mentor drug court program. 2004. Available at: http://state.tn.us/finance/rds/MentorCourtCriteriaandresponsibilities.doc. Accessed January 9, 2008.

[28] Lewis C. Treating incarcerated women: gender matters. Psychiatr Clin North Am 2006; 29(3):773–89.

[29] Kelly TM, Cornelius JR, Clark DB. Psychiatric disorders and attempted suicide among adolescents with substance use disorders. Drug Alcohol Depend 2004;73(1):87–97.

[30] Roman J, Townsend W, Bhati AS. Recidivism rates for drug court graduates: nationally based estimates. 2003. Available at: www.ncjrs.gov/pdffiles1/201229.pdf. Accessed January 1–3, 2008.

[31] Somervell AM, Saylor C, Mao C-L. Public health nurse interventions for women in a dependency drug court [Journal Peer Reviewed Journal]. Public Health Nurs 2005;22(1):59–64.

[32] Eleventh Judicial District of FL. Miami Dade County drug court. 2008. Available at: http:// jud11.flcourts.org/programs_and_services/drug_court.htm. Accessed January 9, 2008.

[33] Office of Criminal Justice Programs. TN drug court annual report 2004–5. 2005. Available at: www.state.tn.us/finance/rds/2005drugctreport.pdf. Accessed January 1–3, 2008.

[34] Office of Criminal Justice Programs. 2005–6 Tennesee drug court annual report. 2006. Available at: http://www.state.tn.us/finance/rds/2005.2006%20Drug%20Court%20Annual% 20Report.doc. Accessed January 1–3, 2008.

[35] Understanding drug abuse and addiction. NIDA InfoFacts 2007 September. Available at: http://www.drugabuse.gov/infofacts/understand.html. Accessed January 2, 2008.

[36] Schiffman RF. Drug and substance use in adolescents [Journal Peer Reviewed Journal]. MCN Am J Matern Child Nurs 2004;29(1):21–7.

[37] Science-based facts on drug abuse and addiction. NIDA InfoFacts. Available at: http:// www.nida.gov/infofacts/Infofaxindex.html. Accessed May 28, 2008.

[38] Speck PM, Connor DP, Small E, et al. Never-served populations: addiction, risk, and health in drug court clients in Memphis TN. Paper presented at the American Public Health Association. Washington, DC. November 3–7, 2007.

[39] Bouffard JA, Smith S. Programmatic, counselor, and client-level comparison of rural versus urban drug court treatment [Journal Peer Reviewed Journal]. Subst Use Misuse 2005;40(3): 321–42.

[40] Sebastian JG. Vulnerability and vulnerable populations: an overview. In: Stanhope M, Lancaster J, editors. Public health nursing: population-centered health care in the community. St. Louis (MO): Mosby; 2008. p. 710–33.

[41] McLellan A. Crime and punishment and treatment: latest findings in the treatment of drug-related offenders [Journal Peer Reviewed Journal Editorial]. J Subst Abuse Treat 2003;25(3): 187–8.

[42] Mertens JR, Lu YW, Parthasarathy S, et al. Medical and psychiatric conditions of alcohol and drug treatment patients in an HMO. Arch Intern Med 2003;163(20):2511–7.

[43] Naegle MA, Richardson H, Morton K. Rehab instead of prison: drug courts provide opportunities for nurse practitioners. Am J Nurs 2004;104(6):58–61.

[44] Smith EM. Race or racism? Addiction in the United States. Ann Epidemiol 1993;3(2): 165–70.

[45] Institute of Medicine. Unequal treatment: confronting racial and ethnic disparities in healthcare. Washington (DC): National Academy Press; 2003.

[46] U.S. Department of Health and Human Services. With understanding and improving health and objectives for improving health. In: Healthy people 2010, vol. 1. 2nd edition. Washington, DC: U.S. Government Printing Office; 2000. Available at: http://www.healthypeople. gov/lhi/factsheet.htm. Accessed May 28, 2008.

[47] Institute of Medicine. American's health-care safety net. Washington, DC: National Academy Press; 2000.

**ELSEVIER
SAUNDERS**

Nurs Clin N Am 43 (2008) 491–496

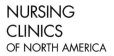

**NURSING
CLINICS**
OF NORTH AMERICA

Index

Note: Page numbers of article titles are in **boldface** type.